Therapeutic Dilemmas for the MRCGP

Dr. Rodger Charlton

BA MPhil MRNZCGP FRCGP
General Practitioner and GP Trainer in the West Midlands and Senior Lecturer in Primary Health Care at Keele University, Staffordshire, UK

and

Dr. John C. Mucklow

MD, FRCP
Consultant Physician and Clinical Pharmacologist at the North Staffordshire Hospital NHS Trust, Stoke-on-Trent and Senior Lecturer in Clinical Pharmacology and Therapeutics at Keele University, Staffordshire, UK

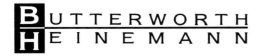
BUTTERWORTH
HEINEMANN

Butterworth-Heinemann
Linacre House, Jordan Hill, Oxford OX2 8DP
225 Wildwood Avenue, Woburn, MA 01801-2041
A division of Reed Educational and Professional Publishing Ltd

 A member of the Reed Elsevier plc group

OXFORD   BOSTON   JOHANNESBURG
MELBOURNE   NEW DELHI   SINGAPORE

First published 1998

© Reed Educational and Professional Publishing Ltd 1998

British Library Cataloguing in Publication Data
A catalogue record for this book is available from the British Library

ISBN 0 7506 2918 5

Typeset by Keyword Typesetting Services Ltd, Wallington, Surrey, England
Printed and bound in Great Britain by Biddles Ltd, Guildford and King's Lynn

Contents

Acknowledgements

This book provides a wide review of therapeutics and some specialized areas of medicine which are rapidly changing. To ensure that the information given to the reader is both accurate and up to date, the chapters have been reviewed by experts, where possible, from the School of Postgraduate Medicine, Keele University. We are most grateful for their comments, sound criticism and advice, and make acknowledgment of their efforts below. (The chapter with which each was concerned is given in brackets.)

Dr.John Gray, Director of the Public Health Laboratory Service, Stoke-on-Trent.

(Antibiotics – when and which?)

Dr. Christina Faull, Medical Director of St.Mary's Hospice, Selly Oak, Birmingham B29 7DA.

(Pain control in palliative care situations in the chapter entitled, Optimal pain relief.)

Dr. Peter T. Dawes, Consultant Rheumatologist, North Staffordshire Rheumatology Centre, Haywood Hospital, Stoke-on-Trent and Senior Clinical Lecturer at the School of Postgraduate Medicine, Keele University.

(Optimal pain relief.)

Dr. Gavin I. Russell, Consultant Nephrologist, North Staffordshire Hospital NHS Trust, Stoke-on-Trent and Senior Lecturer in Medicine, at the School of Postgraduate Medicine, Keele University.

(Lowering blood pressure.)

Dr. Derek G. Waller, Senior Lecturer in Medicine, Southampton General Hospital, Southampton University SO16 6YD.

(Managing Ischaemic Heart Disease.)

Dr. Charles F. A. Pantin, Consultant Physician, North Staffordshire Hospital NHS Trust, Stoke-on-Trent and Senior Lecturer in Respiratory Medicine at the School of Postgraduate Medicine, Keele University.

(Wheezing and Dyspnoea.)

Dr. Warren Lenney, Consultant Respiratory Paediatrician, North Staffordshire Hospital NHS Trust, Stoke-on-Trent and Senior Lecturer at the School of Postgraduate Medicine, Keele University.

(Wheezing and Dyspnoea.)

Dr. John H. B. Scarpello, Consultant Physician, North Staffordshire Hospital NHS Trust, Stoke-on-Trent and Senior Lecturer in Medicine, at the School of Postgraduate Medicine, Keele University.

(Type II Diabetes Mellitus.)

Dr. Charles H. J. Swan, Consultant Physician, Department of Gastroenterology, North Staffordshire Hospital NHS Trust, Stoke-on-Trent and Senior Clinical Lecturer at the School of Postgraduate Medicine, Keele University.

(Gastrointestinal disturbance.)

Miss Sheena Hodgett, Research Fellow and Specialist Registrar, Academic Department of Obstetrics and Gynaecology, North Staffordshire Hospital NHS Trust, Stoke-on-Trent.

(Menstrual regulation and dysfunction.)

Dr. Simon J. Ellis, Consultant Neurologist, North Staffordshire Hospital NHS Trust, Stoke-on-Trent and Senior Clinical Lecturer at the School of Postgraduate Medicine, Keele University.

(Migraine)

Introduction

We intend this textbook to be a learning tool in therapeutics for anyone working in primary care. It aims to meet the needs of general practice registrars who are preparing for the MRCGP examination, and of those wishing to learn more about, or to update their knowledge of, primary care therapeutics. It may also be used by medical undergraduates and others wanting to extend their knowledge in this area.

The title of the book purposely uses the word 'dilemmas', rather than 'controversies'. A dilemma is a position where two or more alternative courses of action are all undesirable. One can argue that all therapies are undesirable because their need stems from disease; in general, people do not wish for ill-health but rather to be well. But the chief reason for using the word 'dilemma' is that no form of drug treatment is ideal for every patient. There is almost always a trade-off to be made between an acceptable risk of unwanted effects and a worthwhile benefit. In many of the clinical scenarios described in the book, the therapeutic options involve a compromise: the preferred option is the 'least worst' rather than the best.

One of the greatest challenges in primary medical practice is that many patients have no identifiable physical disease and yet are ill. In this setting therapeutic dilemmas are often more challenging than in secondary care where the need for treatment is generally more pressing and the use of powerful drugs easier to justify. In general practice, reaching for the prescription pad is often not the answer or the way to facilitate a cure. In the words of the Canadian physician, Sir William Osler (1849-1919):

> The ordering of medicine in any and every malady is no longer regarded as the chief function of the doctor.
> *(Aequanimitas, with Other Addresses, Medicine in the Nineteenth Century.)*

Manual to the textbook

The major part of the text is devoted to common therapeutic dilemmas that illustrate the application of clinical pharmacology to everyday therapeutics. These are intended not only to promote the process of self-directed and problem-based learning, but to follow the structure of the MRCGP examination itself.

Modified essay question (MEQ)

The introduction to each chapter explains the background to the topic and is followed by the dilemma, illustrated through a clinical scenario in a format similar to a modified essay question paper (MEQ) in the MRCGP examination. The MEQ paper has been subject to considerable change over the years and usually consists of 12 questions, each of which will appear on a separate page in the exam itself. Answers should take the form of short notes.

In the exam a separate sheet will be available for each answer. In addition, each page is sent to a different examiner and therefore you should answer each question specifically, even if this involves repetition of part of an earlier answer. (However, for the purposes of space this has not been possible in the book and you should jot your answers on separate sheets of rough paper for practice.)

In the actual exam it is unlikely that questions for the MEQ will be related to each other or on the same subject, but for the purposes of each chapter of this book they are. You are encouraged to consider your own therapeutic management plan before looking up the answer. This approach will also facilitate preparation for the second oral examination. A marking schedule (with a suggested allocation of marks in brackets for each correct answer) is also given to provide a self-assessment of your knowledge, together with a suggested time interval (usually 3 hours) in which to complete your answers. Following many of the answers, a comment section has been added and references from the literature given where appropriate.

Multiple choice questions (MCQS)

A few multiple choice questions (MCQs), similar to those that might appear in the MRCGP examination are provided. In each chapter there are four questions, each of which begins with a statement and is followed by five answers, any or all of which may be true or false. (In the exam marks are not deducted for incorrect answers.) These multiple choice questions are provided to test your knowledge and suggest areas in which further reading is required. Where appropriate a list is given for further reading, making the point that this is not a complete text but rather a learning tool.

Future advances in therapeutics

As advances in therapeutics occur, we hope to revise the book and include up-to-date references.

We hope that you find the book both useful and enjoyable and that it will stimulate and help you in your future medical practice.

1

Antibiotics – when and which?

There has been a great proliferation of antibiotics over the last few years and the two most difficult decisions regarding an antibiotic prescription are:

1. When should an antibiotic be prescribed?
2. If an antibiotic is to be prescribed, which one should it be and how long a course should be taken?

1. When should an antibiotic be prescribed?

This is perhaps the most common and often the most difficult therapeutic dilemma a general practitioner (GP) will face. The decision to prescribe often rests on the patient's circumstances as much as on the clinical justification. Furthermore, this decision has to be balanced against potential unwanted effects (e.g., thrush, gastrointestinal upset and, sometimes, allergy) and the implications of unnecessary antibiotic prescribing (e.g., the emergence of resistant strains, such as MRSA).

The commonest consultation in general practice is the patient with a sore throat or generalized upper respiratory tract infection. Some might see it as the easiest consultation, yet it can be the most difficult. There is no faster way to satisfy a patient than to give them the antibiotic they often request, and if the conscientious and methodical doctor hesitates to prescribe an antibiotic because the illness is self-limiting the patient is sure to remark, 'The last time I had a sore throat, Dr X gave me some penicillin tablets and they magically got rid of it'.

Worse still, the patient may say, 'If it is all the same with you doctor, I would prefer to have an antibiotic'. Plausible and emotive reasons may be given: the patient is due to take exams; go on holiday tomorrow; take their driving test or get married next week. Even our best and well-intentioned attempts at education may not overcome patient expectations.

2. If an antibiotic is to be prescribed, which one should it be and how long a course should be taken?

The rest of the chapter is devoted to this subject and is intended to provide some general guidelines in the prescription of antibiotics.

Modified essay question (MEQ)

(The instructions for the MEQ appear in the manual on page xi.)

Mary, a 22-year-old married lady with a daughter aged 2 years, consults her GP with a 3-day history of sore throat, pain at the sides of her neck, recurrent shivering and feeling unwell. Examination reveals a temperature of 37.5°C, a few lymph nodes in the neck, a fine erythematous rash over her arms and legs and a slight exudate on both tonsils. Mary has attended twice already this year with a history of sore throat and on both occasions has been given a prescription for penicillin V, which appears to have worked well. Her only other medication is the combined oral contraceptive, Ovranette. Coincidentally, she is tearful and tells you that she has been feeling tired all the time for many weeks.

1. *State the differential diagnosis and the possible management
    options.*

Two weeks later Mary consults with a history of dysuria. Fortunately, her sore throat has resolved after a seven day course of penicillin and she feels a lot better in herself.

2. *State your differential diagnosis, the further questions you
    might want to ask, any investigations you might wish to
    perform, and any possible treatment options.*

A year later Mary comes as an emergency to the surgery. She had been gardening a few days earlier and now has an obvious paronychia of one finger with a collection of pus. She is feeling tired and was shivery the night before, and there is reddening around the pus.

3.   Describe the likely diagnosis and your proposed treatment.

Some weeks later Mary calls you at 10.30 pm because her 2-year-old daughter, Natalie, has been crying intermittently and is very hot. (She was well earlier in the day.) She has vomited once and Mary sounds very worried. You decide to visit Natalie at her home and on examination she is alert and smiling intermittently, and has no rash, no signs of meningitis, no abnormality of the ears or throat, a clear chest and no abnormality of the abdomen. As yet, Mary has given her no medication.

4.   Describe the differential diagnosis.

5. *Mary asks if Natalie should have an antibiotic. Describe how you might respond and what therapies are appropriate.*

Natalie improves, but a few weeks later Mary asks you to visit her husband, Simon. She says that she thinks he has 'flu, but she is very worried because he has taken to his bed with a headache, insists on having the curtains shut in the bedroom, and has vomited twice in the last hour. Mary tells you that he has been under a lot of stress lately and his headache is not a new problem. She has measured his temperature and it is 38°C. When you arrive at the house Simon is in bed upstairs in a very dark room. He is leaning over a bowl and vomiting. He cries as you switch the light on. He appears unable to move his neck easily, his pulse rate is 128/min and blood pressure

95/40 mmHg. As you listen to his chest you notice a widespread petechial rash which is becoming purpuric and does not blanch in response to pressure.

6.   What is the differential diagnosis?

7.   What therapeutic action should you take?

Simon recovers from his illness, and Mary and Simon go out to a local restaurant to celebrate their wedding anniversary. Three days later Mary consults you with a history of bloody diarrhoea, abdominal cramps, intermittent fever and feeling generally unwell. Abdominal examination reveals generalized tenderness, active bowel sounds, a pyrexia of 37.5°C; the pulse rate is 88/min and blood pressure 130/80 mmHg. Apparently, Mary had a chicken dish at the restaurant, while Simon had steak and he has had no symptoms.

8.   *What is the differential diagnosis?*

9.   *What is your management plan?*

MEQ answers

(Numbers in brackets refer to the marks you would receive in the MRCGP examination for each part of the answer you mention. Please total your own score to provide self-assessment.)

1. **Differential Diagnosis:**
   Cause of throat infection: viral (1), especially Epstein-Barr virus (1); streptococcal (1).
   Associated rash and fever with any of these (1).

   Management Options:
   Explain the differential diagnosis (1).
   Explain that the problem may settle without antibiotics (1).
   Explain that with the rash the infection may be bacterial and so treatment with an antibiotic may be appropriate, although the benefit is likely to be small (2).
   Suggest that if the problem persists or recurs it would be worth testing for infectious mononucleosis (glandular fever) (2).
   For symptoms of fever and pain it may be worth taking an antipyretic analgesic, such as paracetamol (2).
   Explain that antibiotics can alter the effect of the oral contraceptive pill (1); she should not interrupt this (1) but should use additional contraceptive measures while taking an antibiotic and for a week afterwards (1).
   Discuss whether there are any other reasons in her life for being tired and tearful(1), if this seems appropriate (1).
   If an antibiotic is to be prescribed, penicillin V (phenoxymethyl penicillin) is the most appropriate choice provided there is no history of allergy (2). A dose of 250 mg qds for 7 – 10 days is appropriate (1). If she is allergic to penicillin, the macrolide, erythromycin, would be a suitable alternative (1).

Comment

The dilemma here concerns the uncertainty over whether the infection is bacterial and, if so, whether it warrants use of an antibiotic. The responsible organism cannot reliably be determined from the clinical presentation; throat swabs can also mislead. As there is no reliable diagnostic test that provides a timely answer, it is best to assume that every patient with a sore throat has a bacterial infection. The commonest pathogen is a Group A beta-haemolytic streptococcus (*Strep. pyogenes*). Some strains of this organism produce an exotoxin that causes a diffuse red rash and inflammation of the pharynx and tongue (scarlet fever). In most patients the illness lasts 3–5 days, although the throat and neck can remain tender for up to 2 weeks. The evidence that antibiotic treatment shortens the duration of the illness by 1–2 days at most in those with positive cultures is inconsistent, neither is it clear whether antibiotics prevent the suppurative complications of a sore throat, such as sinusitis and otitis media. As for the immunological sequelae, post-streptococcal glomerulonephritis and rheumatic fever, their incidence in developed countries has been falling since well before the discovery of antibiotics, probably because of a change in the virulence of the organism, and only one in five GPs in Britain is likely ever to see a patient with either of these conditions.

If the benefit of prescribing an antibiotic is so marginal, one must also consider the disadvantages. The incidence of allergic reactions to penicillin in general practice is about 1 in 25 patients treated, although a serious reaction is much less likely to occur (1.5–4 cases per 10,000 patients, with 2 deaths per 100,000). Whereas antibiotic resistance is not at present a major problem in general practice in the UK, a report from Finland in 1992 revealed a worrying increase in the number of streptococcal strains resistant to erythromycin; before this report was published erythromycin was being preferred in 10% of Finnish patients infected with Group A streptococcus. It is worth remembering that Group A streptococcus can also cause conditions more serious than a sore throat, such as skin sepsis, endocarditis and meningitis. The future prevalence of antibiotic resistance can be reduced by avoiding unnecessary use of antibiotics, and by selecting them logically and consistently. Adults with sore throats are quite willing to accept an explanation and symptomatic treatment (e.g., analgesic, saline gargle) as an alternative to an antibiotic, even in painful upper respiratory conditions.

2. **Differential Diagnosis:**
   Cystitis (1).
   Urethritis, due to infection with *Chlamydia trachomatis*, *Neisseria gonorrhoeae*, or *Herpes simplex* virus (3).
   Vaginitis, due to Candida or *Trichomonas vaginalis* (2) (following use of an antibiotic) (1).

Further questions:
Is there frequency, haematuria, loin/back pains or fever? (4).
Is there discharge, bleeding, pruritus, or dyspareunia? (4).

Examination:
Look for suprapubic tenderness, inflammation of vulva, vagina and cervix, and herpetic lesions (3).

Possible Investigations:
Mid-stream Specimen of Urine (MSU) to be sent for culture and sensitivity, particularly in the case of recurrent or persistent cystitis (1).
High Vaginal Swab (HVS) to be sent for culture and sensitivity (1).
Cervical or urethral swab for chlamydia and gonococcal culture (2).

Treatment Options:
Await results of investigations (1).
Advise plenty of fluids (1).
Suggest drinks, such as Barley Water, that will alkalinize the urine (1).
For suspected Urinary Tract Infection (UTI) prescribe trimethoprim 200 mg bd for 3 days (1) (Advice regarding the oral contraceptive pill and the prescription of antibiotics as detailed previously (1)).
For suspected vaginal thrush prescribe clotrimazole pessaries (1), with clotrimazole cream if there are any external symptoms (1), and treatment for her husband if appropriate (1).
Review if her symptoms do not settle (1).

Comment

Cystitis in young women is usually caused by *Escherichia coli*, less often by *Staphylococcus saprophyticus*, *Proteus sp.* or *Klebsiella sp.* The risk of infection is increased by sexual intercourse, the use of a diaphragm and spermicide, delayed postcoital micturition, and a recent urinary tract infection. All should have a short course of empirical antibiotic therapy. A three-day course of treatment is sufficient except for the following categories, in whom a seven-day course is justified:

Age > 65;
Pregnant;
Diabetic;
Symptoms for longer than a week;
Recent UTI;
History of UTI caused by resistant organisms;
Use of diaphragm.

The drug of choice is trimethoprim on grounds of efficacy, safety and cost. Although some strains of *E. coli* (5-15%) are resistant, the proportion is not high enough to consider discarding this drug at

present. Alternatives include nitrofurantoin, cephalexin and nor-
floxacin, in order of increasing cost. Resistance among *E. coli* to
amoxycillin is now unacceptably high. It is not cost effective to
routinely send urine samples for culture and dipstick testing for
nitrite/leucocyte esterase is unreliable; urine culture should be
reserved for those with recurrent or persistent infection.

The explanation that is invoked to explain instances of contraceptive failure resulting from the interaction between antibiotics
and the oral contraceptive involves gut flora in an enterohepatic
cycle. Conjugated ethinyl oestradiol is excreted via the biliary tree
into the gut where it is hydrolysed by gut flora, allowing the hormone to be reabsorbed, so the contraceptive effect is sustained.
Elimination of the gut flora by antimicrobials reduces the extent
of this hydrolysis, so the hormone is eliminated more rapidly.
Considering the volume of antibiotics prescribed, contraceptive failure in these circumstances is surprisingly rare, perhaps because of
differences among women in the proportion of ethinyl oestradiol
undergoing conjugation (as opposed to hydroxylation), and among
gut bacteria in their susceptibility to the antibiotic used. Most
reported instances of contraceptive failure have occurred after
treatment with ampicillin, amoxycillin and tetracycline, but precautionary measures should not be confined to the use of these drugs.

3. **Diagnosis**
    Acute staphylococcal infection (1).

    Treatment
    Incision and drainage of pus (1).
    Advice regarding the wound & dressings (1).
    Ensure she is up to date with tetanus immunizations (1).
    Prescription for flucloxacillin if there is no penicillin allergy (1),
    otherwise co-trimoxazole or cephalexin (erythromycin is not
    effective against all strains of staphylococci) (1).
    Advice regarding the oral contraceptive pill and the prescrip-
    tion of antibiotics as detailed previously (1).
    Review in two days or earlier if there is a deterioration (1).

4. Upper Respiratory Tract Infection (URTI): viral (1); bacterial
    (1).
    Viral Infection, e.g., chicken pox (1).

5. Explain that the most likely cause of her symptoms is viral (1)
    and that it would be most appropriate to administer an analge-

sic and antipyretic, such as a suspension of paracetamol (1) (120 mg/5 ml - 5 ml 6 hourly as required) (1).

Ensure that Mary understands that antibiotics are unlikely to make any difference at this stage in the absence of signs of a bacterial infection (1) and may have unwanted effects, such as diarrhoea. (1).

Ensure that she understands when to consult again should Natalie not improve (1). For example, if Natalie develops a severe earache or chesty cough (1), or if she becomes worse with continuous vomiting, a rash and extreme lethargy (1) when illnesses such as meningitis should be considered (1).

6. Acute infection (1), most likely meningitis (1), and possibly meningococcal septicaemia (1).

7. Injection of intravenous penicillin G 1200 mg (2 megaUnit) (1). Organize immediate admission to hospital (1).
    Treatment of close contacts with an antibiotic, such as rifampicin, as directed by local microbiologist (1).

Comment

Acute community-acquired bacterial meningitis can be caused by *Haemophilus influenzae* type b (uncommon in adults aged 18–50), *Neisseria meningitidis*, or *Streptococcus pneumoniae*. The commonest features (in c. 85%) are fever, headache, meningism, and clouding of consciousness. The clinical presentation is seldom a guide to the causative agent, although 50% of patients with meningococcaemia, with or without meningitis, present with a prominent rash, primarily apparent on the extremities, typically erythematous and macular at first but evolving into a petechial phase with later coalescence into purpura.

This is a diagnosis where speed is paramount. Ideally, patients with suspected bacterial meningitis should have their cerebrospinal fluid (CSF) examined within 30 minutes, before the initiation of appropriate antimicrobial therapy, but this is seldom practicable. Because mortality increases with every minute's delay the priority is to start antibiotic therapy within an hour of clinical diagnosis, using drugs that will cover all likely causative organisms. Increasing resistance to chloramphenicol among strains of *H. influenzae* and (to a lesser extent) to penicillin and chloramphenicol among strains of *Strep. pneumoniae* has led many hospitals to use ceftriaxone as empirical antimicrobial therapy in adults. But ceftriaxone has to be given by IV infusion, and in the community a bolus IV injection of benzylpenicillin is equally satisfactory as a first line measure. In patients who have experienced an anaphylactic reaction (nothing less) to penicillin in the past, cefotaxime 1–2 g IV would be appropriate. If possible, a blood culture should be taken before giving the injection.

Once a diagnosis of meningococcal meningitis has been confirmed, treatment of close contacts with rifampicin, as discussed with the Consultant in Communicable Disease Control, is intended to eliminate nasopharyngeal carriage of the pathogenic strain; the patient probably acquired the infection from an asymptomatic carrier with whom they came into contact. It is simpler to treat all contacts than to hunt for the responsible carrier. In local outbreaks (e.g., in schools, barracks or prisons) protection of contacts from infection may require vaccination. At present, vaccines are available only against groups A and C meningococci, whereas in the developed world group B meningococcus is the most prevalent. However, group B vaccines are under trial and may soon be available.

8. **Gastroenteritis** (1):
   Viral
   Bacterial: campylobacter (1) or salmonella (1).

9. Arrange to obtain a stool culture (1).
   Encourage increased fluid intake (1).
   Consider antibiotics, such as erythromycin, as campylobacter is the most likely cause (2).
   Arrange to review the patient (1) particularly if the situation deteriorates (1).
   Review the situation when the stool culture results are available (1).
   Notify the Consultant in Communicable Disease Control of suspected food poisoning (1).
   Perform a further stool culture once Mary is better (1).

Comment

Viral causes of gastroenteritis in adults include rotavirus (groups A–C) (uncommon), Norwalk and related viruses, and adenovirus, the latter being more likely to affect the immunocompromised. The incubation period for rotavirus infection is 24–48 hours and the illness presents suddenly with watery diarrhoea and vomiting, often preceded by coryza and a cough. The incubation period for Norwalk virus infection is similar, but nausea and vomiting are much more prominent than diarrhoea.

Salmonella gastroenteritis has an incubation period of 16–48 hours and presents with vomiting and diarrhoea; fever is not invariable.

Campylobacter is now the commonest bacterial cause of gastro-enteritis in most developed countries. Infection occurs commonly after eating undercooked meat, particularly poultry, and is more common during the summer months. The incubation period is 3–5 days and the illness presents with malaise, cramping abdominal pain and loose, watery stools that may become bloody. Stool culture is diagnostic and most patients recover within a few days with fluid replacement alone. Antibiotic therapy is necessary only if symptoms are prolonged or severe. Erythromycin is the drug of choice, but in patients who have tolerated this drug poorly in the past, ciprofloxacin is the preferred alternative and will also cover salmonella.

(Total available marks = 90.)

Further reading

Anon. (1996). The most cost-effective options for treating UTIs still to be established. *Drugs & Therapy Perspectives,* **8(10)**, 13–16.

Back, D.J., Grimmer, S.F.M., Orme, M.L'E, Proudlove, C., Mann, R.D., and Breckenridge, A.M. (1998). Evaluation of Committee on Safety of Medicines yellow card reports on oral contraceptive-drug interactions with anticonvulsants and antibiotics. *Br. J. Clin. Pharmacol.,* **25**, 527–532.

Bannister, B. (1996). Skin and soft tissue infections. *Med. Internat.,* **24(8)**, 57–63.

Dagnelie, C.F., van der Graaf, Y., de Melker, R.A. and Touw-Otten, F.W.M.M. (1996). Do patients with sore throats benefit from penicillin? A randomised double-blind placebo-controlled clinical trial with penicillin V in general practice. *Br. J. Gen. Pract.,* **46**, 589–593.

Desselberger, U. (1996). Viral gastroenteritis. *Med. Internat.,* **24(8)**, 52–54.

Kelsey, M.C., Kouloumas, G.A., Lamport, P.A., and Davis, C.L. (1996). Relation between general practitioners' prescribing of antibacterial drugs and their use of laboratory tests. *Br. Med. J.,* **313**, 922.

Lever, A.M.L. (1996). Meningitis. *Med. Internat.,* **24(8)**, 34–38.

Little, P.S., Williamson, I., Shvartzman, P. and Rubin, P.C. (1994). Controversies in management. Are antibiotics appropriate for sore throats? *Br. Med. J.,* **309**, 1010–1012.

Martin, M.J., and Griffin, G.E. (1996). Bacterial gastroenteritis. *Med. Internat.,* **24(8)**, 47–51.

O'Brien, T.F. (1992). Global surveillance of antibiotic resistance. *N. Engl. J. Med.,* **326**, 339–340.

Pollard, A.J., and Booy, R. (1997). Editorial: Keeping the meningococcus out of the media. *Br. J. Gen. Pract.*, **47**, 201-202.

Ross Russell, R. (1996). Streptococcal and staphylococcal infections. *Med. Internat.*, **24(8)**, 68–70.

Stamm, W.E., and Hooton, T.M. (1993). Management of urinary tract infections in adults. *N Engl J Med*, **329**, 1328–1334.

Tunkel, A.R., and Schield, W.M. (1995). Acute bacterial meningitis. *Lancet*, **346**, 1675–1680.

Wyatt, T.D., Passmore, C.M., Morrow, N.C., and Reilly, P.M. (1990). Antibiotic prescribing: the need for a policy in general practice. *Br. Med. J.*, **300**, 441–444.

Multiple choice questions (MCQ)

(The following four statements are each followed by five answers. Please indicate whether each is true or false.)

1. **The following are true statements:**

   a) Amoxycillin is the drug of choice for infectious mono-nucleosis.
   b) Tetracycline is a good choice for otitis media in children.
   c) Flucloxacillin is a useful antibiotic for staphylococcal infections.
   d) Chlorpromazine can have an antihelmintic effect.
   e) Ciprofloxacin is a 4-quinolone.

2. **The following antibiotics are available for oral use:**

   a) Macrolides.
   b) Aminoglycosides.
   c) Cephalosporins.
   d) Chloramphenicol.
   e) Penicillin G.

3. **The following are useful antifungal agents:**

   a) Mebendazole.
   b) Clotrimazole.
   c) Metronidazole.
   d) Vancomycin.
   e) Co-trimoxazole.

4. **The following statements about antimicrobial agents are true:**

   a) Flucloxacillin is effective against methicillin-resistant *Staphylococcus aureus*.
   b) Augmentin contains ampicillin and clavulanic acid.
   c) Topical clindamycin can be used in acne.
   d) Clindamycin can cause pseudomembranous colitis.
   e) Nalidixic acid is useful in urinary tract infections.

Answers overleaf

MCQ answers

(A maximum total of 20 marks are available.)

1. F,F,T,T,T.
2. T,F,T,T,F.
3. F,T,F,F,F.
4. F,F,T,T,T.

Optimal pain relief

This chapter examines the management of a variety of pain problems that are commonly encountered in primary care and provides some general principles concerning the use of analgesics. In other chapters pain associated with gastrointestinal disturbance, ischaemic heart disease, menstruation and migraine are discussed, and you should refer to the appropriate chapter for these particular problems. Pain is a subjective symptom and varies among individual patients suffering with the same conditions. Sometimes, patients have great difficulty describing the pain that they are experiencing.

Let a sufferer try to describe a pain in the head to a doctor and language runs at once dry.

(Virginia Woolf)

The description of an unpleasant distressing sensation or sensations, in one or several parts of the body, vary according to the sufferer's reaction to them.

But pain is perfect miserie,
the worst of evils,
and excessive,
overturnes all patience.

(Milton, *Paradise Lost.*)

The causes of pain are complex and not purely physical. Pain can be modified by coexistent psychological and emotional processes. To provide adequate analgesia, the first priority is adequate communication: explanation alone can raise the pain threshold and tolerance. It is important also to explain that analgesia may not abolish pain altogether, but may make it more tolerable.

There are several dilemmas in the management of pain. The doctor must first decide whether the pain has an 'organic cause'. Is the patient using the symptom as a means of attracting attention or of securing treatment with an opiate? If the pain is organic, what is its nature? A confident diagnosis simplifies the choice of agent whereas uncertainty may justify empirical treatment, the response to which is itself a diagnostic aid.

How severe is the pain? It is important to ensure that the drug and dosage chosen afford some, if not complete, relief, while at the same time avoiding unwanted effects that might compromise both pain relief and future management.

The final part of the chapter examines the use of analgesics and in particular, opiates, and their role in patients who are terminally ill and in pain.

Modified essay question (MEQ)

(The instructions for the MEQ appear in the manual on page xi.)

Sandy, a 33-year-old man presents with a three-day history of lower back pain after lifting some heavy objects in his garden. The pain is over his lumbar spine and does not radiate, there are no associated parasthesiae, he has no disturbance in the function of his bowels or bladder, and examination is unremarkable, except for some minor discomfort on spinal movement of the lower back and evidence of muscle spasm. He describes the pain as a constant dull ache, worse on movement. As yet, he has taken no medication and wishes your advice. A diagnosis of lumbago is made.

1. What analgesics might you suggest that he uses and why?

Sandy's mother is aged 70 years and lives with Sandy and his wife. She has been suffering with decreasing mobility as a result of osteoarthritis in her knees and hips. She is not overweight and has been trying to take regular exercise. She seldom visits the surgery but attends later in the week because the co-proxamol tablets she has been taking have not been sufficient to alleviate the pain she has been getting. The pain is worst when she gets up in the morning and examination reveals a slight limitation of hip movements and considerable crepitus in both knees. She consults you to ask if there is any other medication that she can take.

2. What therapeutic alternatives are available?

Sandy's wife, Amanda, books an appointment with you for her 6-year-old son, Tom. He has been complaining of intermittent tummy pains for the last week. There has been no history of diarrhoea or vomiting. You inquire about his appetite to be told, 'He never eats, just picks all the time and will only eat "junk food"'. The pain has not stopped him from going to school, but last night he awoke with pain and Amanda says, 'I don't think he is putting it on doctor, I just don't know what is wrong. Can you help?'.

3.   Describe your management of Tom.

A few weeks later Amanda rings you at 10 pm. She sounds upset and asks if you could visit straight away as for the last hour Sandy has been holding his abdomen, crying with pain and unable to keep still. He has vomited once and has had no previous similar episode.

You visit Sandy straight away and find, as you try to examine his abdomen, that he is unable to keep still. Examination reveals no abnormality other than tenderness in the left loin. Normal bowel sounds are present. His pulse is 96/min and regular and his blood pressure is 150/95 mmHg. By coincidence, he has passed a urine specimen which yields blood (+ +) on testing.

4.   *What is the most likely diagnosis and why? What is your treatment plan?*

Five years later, Amanda finds a lump in her right breast. A needle biopsy reveals a poorly differentiated carcinoma of the breast and at mastectomy there are several affected axillary lymph glands. The prognosis is poor and an early menopause is induced through ovarian oblation in an attempt to reduce her oestrogen production. She also has a course of local radiotherapy but elects not to have chemotherapy. Four months after operation, it becomes apparent that there are bony metastases throughout her skeleton and she has evidence of ascites and an enlarged liver. Her main problem is of generalized pain and resultant immobility.

5.   *How would you choose appropriate analgesia and what might you start with, assuming that Amanda has tried no analgesics yet? What are the likely side-effects?*

6. *Amanda responds moderately well to the analgesics you have prescribed. Can you suggest any adjuvant therapies that might augment the effect of the analgesics prescribed?*

7. *Two months later Amanda is on large doses of opioids, but pain is still a problem and she is asking about non-pharmacological methods of pain relief. What advice might you give her?*

MEQ answers

(Numbers in brackets refer to the marks you would receive in the MRCGP examination for each part of the answer you mention. Please total your own score to provide self-assessment.)

1. Paracetamol 1 g 4–6 hourly as required, to maximum 4 g daily (1). This drug is unlikely to cause unwanted effects (1) and can be purchased over the counter for less than a prescription charge (1).

   If this is ineffective, compound analgesics containing paracetamol and a weak opioid may be tried, such as co-proxamol, co-codamol or co-dydramol, which also contain dextropropoxyphene, codeine and dihydrocodeine respectively. Sandy should be informed that these may lead to constipation and he will need to take a laxative regularly (3).

   There is another group of drugs which may be more effective: the non-steroidal anti-inflammatory drugs (NSAIDs) (1). These have both an analgesic effect and an anti-inflammatory effect, which may be beneficial in low back pain (2). However, caution should be exercised as they have two important unwanted effects. First, NSAIDs can cause indigestion (1) and so should be taken with or after food; second, and less commonly, they can precipitate or worsen bronchospasm (1). These side-effects are particularly pertinent in patients who suffer with dyspepsia and asthma respectively (2). These drugs should be avoided in patients with gastrointestinal ulceration or bleeding, or with a history of hypersensitivity to aspirin or other NSAIDs. Examples of two NSAIDs that can be purchased over the counter are soluble aspirin 600 mg six hourly or ibuprofen 400 mg three times daily (2).

   It seems reasonable to start with these alternatives and consider the use of stronger analgesics if these are unsuccessful (1).

Comment

Back pain is the commonest cause of work absenteeism in those aged under 45 years. The aims of treatment are to relieve pain and stiffness, to reduce inflammation (if present) and to preserve function. Current thinking has moved away from advising rest and lying on a firm surface to advising a return to normal activities as soon as is practically possible. Regular paracetamol is the best tolerated drug, but also the least effective. Whereas there is no evidence that compound analgesics in single doses work better than paracetamol alone, regular dosing may afford greater relief in individual patients, perhaps because the weak opioid component is more slowly eliminated than paracetamol, and so accumulates. Co-dydramol (dihydrocodeine 10 mg, paracetamol 500 mg) is more effective than co-codamol (codeine 8 mg, paracetamol 500 mg), which is more effective than co-proxamol (d-propoxyphene 32.5 mg, paracetamol 325 mg). The opioid content of these agents is modest and co-codamol 8/500 can be purchased over the counter, whereas the stronger 30/500 formulation (e.g., Solpadol, Tylex) is prescription-only.

NSAIDs are likely to be more effective than paracetamol only if inflammation is contributing to the pain by causing the release of prostaglandins that heighten the sensitivity of nerve endings. Aspirin, at a daily dosage less than 3 g, and ibuprofen, at a daily dosage of 1200 mg, may not have sufficient anti-inflammatory effect to make a difference, but treatment should start at these dosages to minimize unwanted effects.

Peptic ulceration and gastrointestinal bleeding are less common in younger adults than in the elderly, but NSAIDs should be reserved for those whose pain is resistant to other measures and who have no recent history of ulceration. Hypersensitivity to aspirin and other NSAIDs is uncommon and affects only 5–10% of asthmatics; those affected will usually have coincident sinusitis, nasal polyps and eosinophilia, though sensitivity is more common in adult-onset non-allergic asthma than in allergic asthma. Most asthmatics will experience no ill-effects from symptomatic use of aspirin and other NSAIDs. If hypersensitivity is suspected it should be established by formal challenge under specialist supervision; patients should not be denied access to an important group of drugs without clear evidence that they are contraindicated.

2. Stronger analgesics, such as co-codamol or co-dydramol, may be considered (2). However, the patient should be warned in case constipation results. Alternatively, if she has no upper gastrointestinal problems a long acting NSAID may be considered (1), for example, diclofenac 100 mg slow release capsules (1).

    Other therapeutic alternatives include physiotherapy (1), hydrotherapy (1) or intra-articular steroid injections to settle joint inflammation, and so pain (2).

Comment

Whereas there is no evidence that compound analgesics are superior to paracetamol alone in osteoarthritis, some patients prefer them. Stronger opioids should be avoided; if they have to be considered, a reassessment of the cause(s) of the pain is necessary. There is little evidence that NSAIDs are superior to paracetamol, even when an anti-inflammatory dose (e.g., ibuprofen 2400 mg/day) is used. Although some patients find that NSAIDs afford better symptom control, these drugs should be reserved for those resistant to other measures. It should be remembered that up to 40% of patients will have a placebo response for up to six weeks.

Osteoarthritis is commonest in women, in the very age group that tolerates NSAIDs least well. Gastrointestinal complications, fluid retention, interstitial nephritis and serious drug interactions result in significant morbidity and mortality.

Where pain is confined to one or two joints, it is worth considering intra-articular or peri-articular injection of corticosteroid before introducing an NSAID. Transient symptomatic relief may be appreciable and injections can be repeated, if necessary, up to three times a year without ill-effect. More frequent injections can result in a neuropathic (Charcot) joint.

If an NSAID has to be used, it is best to add it to existing analgesia (rather than to substitute) and to use the smallest effective dosage regularly, reassessing the need for treatment and trying to reduce dosage whenever possible. Offer occasional courses and avoid repeat prescriptions. NSAIDs differ in their propensity to cause gastrointestinal bleeding and perforation; ibuprofen, naproxen and diclofenac are among the safest, whereas longer-acting drugs, such as azapropazone, are much less safe. Newer NSAIDs such as nabumetone and meloxicam may have a better safety profile, but are more expensive. Attempting to prevent gastric ulceration by prophylactic use of misoprostol can cause troublesome gastric bloating and diarrhoea and is not cost-effective, unless used selectively in those with a history of peptic ulceration and the frail elderly, who are most at risk.

3. Examination (1) of Tom is mandatory and this should include an initial assessment of whether he is alert and playful, or ill and lethargic. A full examination of his throat should be made (1) to exclude swollen, tender lymph glands in his neck (1) which can be associated with swollen, painful mesenteric glands (mesenteric adenitis) (1). If pyrexia is also present his ears should be examined and his chest auscultated to exclude a

source of infection (1). Abdominal examination should be performed (1) to exclude acute abdominal conditions such as appendicitis (1). Finally, if the diagnosis is still in doubt a specimen of urine should be analysed and sent for culture and sensitivity as a urinary tract infection can present with abdominal pain in children (1).

If one can be confident that serious pathology will not be masked by treatment, paracetamol elixir may be prescribed at a dose of 250 mg six hourly (1). Finally, Tom's mother should bring him for review if the pain persists or worsens (1).

4. Ureteric colic should be suspected (1) with the sudden onset, the history of severe colic, the presence of blood in the urine and no other obvious abnormality (4). First, his pain should be treated, and two analgesics may be considered. An intramuscular injection of the opioid, pethidine 100 mg (1), should be effective but this may have central nervous system side-effects (1). You should explain that the pain will gradually settle with this but that it may make him drowsy (1). A useful alternative is the NSAID, diclofenac 75 mg, which can be given either by intramuscular injection or as a suppository. Second, arrangements should be made to investigate the problem in hospital (1) where an IVP (intravenous pyelogram) can be carried out (1) looking for a residual stone in the upper urinary tract.

5. The World Health Organisation has described an 'analgesic ladder' (1) and treatment should progress through the following three steps according to the type and severity of pain (1).

The first step is administration of a non-opioid, such as paracetamol (1). Its singular advantage is an almost complete absence of side-effects (1); up to 4 g can be given daily in divided doses. Furthermore, it is available in tablets or soluble form, or as 125 mg suppositories. Paracetamol is also useful as an antipyretic and as a treatment for headache, which often responds poorly to opioids. All other analgesics have potential or inevitable side-effects. The other important non-opioid analgesics are the NSAIDs (1). These are particularly useful for bone pain that is resistant to paracetamol (1). The least toxic is ibuprofen, which should be taken with food to minimize gastric side-effects (1).

For pain uncontrolled by non-opioids, the second step in the ladder is to add a weak opioid (1), such as dextropropoxyphene, codeine phosphate or dihydrocodeine tartrate. Given in combination with paracetamol, rather than alone, they will give additive analgesia (1) with fewer dose-related opioid side-effects (1). Co-codamol 30/500 should be preferred to the 8/500 formulation (1). All three can cause drowsiness, nausea and constipation; the patient should be warned about these (3) and given a prophylactic stimulant laxative.

When stronger opioids are needed to control pain, morphine or another strong opioid (2), the third step on the analgesic ladder, should be considered. The starting dose is chosen according to the previous analgesia used (1). For example, 5-10mg of morphine may be given if a weak analgesic, such as co-proxamol, was being used, or 10–20 mg if a stronger analgesic, such as co-dydramol, was being used (2). The dose chosen should be given by mouth, if the patient's condition allows, every four hours (1). After the first 24 hours, if the pain has not been completely relieved, the four-hourly dose should be increased by 30–50% and titrated upwards against the pain daily (3).

Initially, morphine should be given as elixir (e.g., Oramorph) or conventional tablets (e.g., Sevredol) because sustained-release morphine does not achieve its peak effect for four-and-a-half hours (2).

Once pain has been prevented and no breakthrough has occurred for 24 hours, sustained-release tablets/suspension can be substituted if the patient wants (1). The daily dosage should be the same as the total requirement for morphine during the previous 24 hours, given as a modified release formulation every 12 (e.g., MST) or 24 (e.g., MXL) hours (2); give the first dose of sustained-release morphine together with the last dose of Oramorph/Sevredol and prescribe 'as required' doses of Oramorph equivalent to 1/6th of the 24 hour requirement (2). There is no upper limit to the dose of morphine: the right dose is that required to keep the patient pain free yet conscious (1). Morphine reduces intestinal motility, so a stimulant laxative must also be prescribed (1). Once a 12 or 24 hour regimen is established (1), it should be reviewed daily and increased (maintaining the same dose interval) if extra doses of Oramorph have been required (2).

For many reasons a patient may not be able to take medication by mouth and a parenteral route might need to be considered (1). It is important to avoid painful IM injections and a continuous subcutaneous infusion of diamorphine using a syringe driver should be preferred (1). To calculate the dose requirement, divide the total daily dose of morphine by 3 and infuse over 24 hours (1). The injection site should be changed every 2-3 days if necessary to avoid skin irritation (1).

Finally, fentanyl, which is used by injection for intra-operative analgesia, has recently been introduced in a transdermal drug delivery system as a self-adhesive patch which is changed every 72 hours (2). This comes in four strengths, 25, 50, 75 or 100 micrograms per hour (1). When substituting transdermal fentanyl for morphine, once pain is controlled, one 25 microgram per hour patch gives approximately the same analgesia as 90 mg morphine given over 24 hours (1). Fentanyl patches are expensive, but they may be useful in patients who cannot tolerate morphine, or who are unable to take oral morphine and find a syringe driver impractical or unacceptable (2).

Comment

Analgesics may be divided into three categories; non-opioid, weak opioids and strong opioids. An opioid is any naturally occurring or synthetic drug that is specifically antagonised by naloxone.

A useful principle to apply when prescribing for terminally-ill patients is that the total number of drugs given should be as few as possible, the prescription being regularly reviewed and rationalized. The patient at home should be supplied with a sheet or card clearly stating which tablet is to be taken and when. A Medidose Pill Container should be considered.

Summary: Analgesic Ladder
   Non-opioids
   paracetamol
   NSAIDs for bone pain
   Weak opioids and non-opioids
   co-proxamol
   co-codamol
   co-dydramol
   Strong opioids
   morphine
   diamorphine (heroin)
   fentanyl

When prescribing those drugs in step three of the analgesic ladder, it is important to overcome the notion that there is a dose limit. There is little risk of addiction or tolerance. This is borne out in clinical practice with the terminally-ill, who do not take opioids for their euphoric effect and can be maintained on the same dose for many weeks. They seldom experience withdrawal when these drugs are stopped if they are no longer required. Any need for a higher dose is likely to be due to increased pain because of the natural progression of cancer. This information must be fully shared with the patient.

The prescriber must also be reassured that oral morphine has been repeatedly shown in clinical practice not to depress respiration, even in patients with chest disease, despite a theoretical risk. (Pain is the physiological antagonist of opioids' depressant effect.) This also applies to parenteral morphine, provided the patient has already been given oral morphine. It is often beneficial where dyspnoea is a problem.

The dose should be increased gradually; a large initial dose should be necessary only where pain is overwhelming. Morphine should never be reserved for use as a last resort. It must be given whenever pain is severe enough to warrant this therapeutic approach. Nor is it true that morphine can never be stopped; pain can suddenly be relieved, for example, following a nerve block.

A conversion table for the different strong opioid preparations.
The following are approximate equivalents:

90 mg modified release morphine twice daily (MST Continus, Napp) or 180 mg modified release morphine once daily (MXL, Napp).

30 mg oral morphine solution 4 hourly.

20 mg oral diamorphine solution 4 hourly.

10 mg of subcutaneous diamorphine over four hours (60mg over 24 hours).

50 micrograms of transdermal fentanyl per hour.

The use of opioids always causes side effects and a balance needs to be struck between adequate pain relief and tolerable side-effects. These drugs always cause constipation and this should be routinely countered by giving an aperient that is both a stimulant and a stool softener (e.g. co-danthramer, or senna with lactulose).

Nausea and even vomiting may be a problem initially and this can be treated with an anti-emetic, such as haloperidol 1.5–3.0 mg 12 hourly. Like drowsiness, nausea will quickly wear off after a few days.

Drowsiness and confusion may occur in a patient whose effective daily dose of morphine has been ascertained, but who undergoes palliative radiotherapy or chemotherapy. The resultant reduction in tumour size and pain reduces the extent to which drowsiness is countered by pain, and the dose of morphine can be reduced.

Great care is necessary in patients with renal or hepatic failure, where a smaller dose of morphine is required; it can often be reduced by 50%. Similar care is required in the elderly.

6. Amitriptyline (1) is particularly useful where pain is neuropathic or has become persistent or chronic, and is often effective at a much smaller dose (e.g., 25–50 mg daily) than would be necessary to treat depression (1). Carbamazepine (1) may be considered where there is nerve irritation Where anxiety is a problem, anxiolytics, such as diazepam or chlorpromazine may be valuable (2). Corticosteroids, as prednisolone or dexamethasone are particularly useful in patients with pain arising from nerve compression or raised intracranial pressure (2).

Comment

At any step of the analgesic ladder, an adjuvant to the analgesia may be added. An adjuvant is any drug whose primary indication is other than for pain. It may enhance the effect of an analgesic, or become analgesic itself in certain conditions. For example, pain arising from nerve irritation may respond to the anticonvulsant, carbamazepine, or the tricyclic antidepressant, amitriptyline.

To control pain it is sometimes necessary to control the associated anxiety with psychotropic drugs, such as chlorpromazine and diazepam. Chlorpromazine may be especially beneficial through its anti-emetic effect if nausea or vomiting are present. Diazepam is also useful for associated muscle spasm. Both can cause drowsiness. In the long-term, spending time with the patient, listening to their concerns and, if available, recommending a patient support group may be more beneficial. The advice of a specialist palliative care team can be particularly useful in this situation.

Studies have been performed using corticosteroids as adjuvant analgesics. How they work in this situation is largely unknown but their effects can be dramatic. They are not beneficial to all patients, but are worth considering in patients with persistent pain as a result of advanced cancer. Their additional advantages are that they create a feeling of well-being, and improve appetite and so quality of life. However, their unwanted effects can be severe, and include skin fragility (leading to bed-sores), candidiasis, infection, peptic ulceration and hyperglycaemia. Dexamethasone is the drug of choice as it has little mineralocorticoid effect and is seven times as potent as prednisolone, so fewer tablets are necessary. A suggested starting dosage is 4 mg twice daily, reduced or increased according to response. Where bony metastases are present, radiotherapy may alleviate bone pain.

7. The cause of the pain should be reassessed; it may have changed (1). Many members of the health care team should be involved in treating pain as well as the doctor and nurse. For example, a counsellor, psychologist or member of the clergy (3). An occupational therapist (1) may be able to improve quality of life by providing aids and a physiotherapist (1) can help by increasing mobility, thereby relieving the pain caused by stiffness.
    Complementary therapies include hypnotherapy (1), hydrotherapy (1), homeopathy (1), massage (1), aromatherapy (1), reflexology (1), special diets (1) and faith healing (1). Two therapies commonly available from pain clinics or specialists are transcutaneous electrical nerve stimulation (TENS) (1) and acupuncture (1).

Comment

Pain is not a single entity. It has many causes and these should be considered and reviewed at each encounter. Sometimes a simple measure may succeed where intolerable doses of morphine have failed. Pain control may prove elusive for reasons which are not necessarily physical. There may be a failure of communication or assessment. Review may be too infrequent to treat the recurrence of pain and the patient may have unresolved emotional, psychological or spiritual conflicts. Pain should not be seen as an insurmountable challenge.

TENS can be used at pulsed low frequency (1–2 Hz) for neuropathic pain or at continuous high frequency (40–150 Hz) for somatic pain due to tissue damage. Initially, as many as 80% of patients may respond and there are few side-effects. It is applied through two small electrodes on the skin, connected to a portable battery-operated stimulator. However, after a year of treatment, only 35% may be responding.

Acupuncture produces a mildly painful stimulus by insertion of a fine needle at carefully defined acupuncture points. It can be highly effective in relieving pain in certain patients but may not be suitable for all. There has been little rigorous assessment of its clinical value.

No patient should have to die in pain. If the pharmacological measures outlined fail, referral to a specialist in palliative medicine should be considered. There may also be a role for the anaesthetist and the use of nerve blocks.

(Total possible marks = 112.)

Further reading

Anon. (1996). Opioid use for terminal care can be improved. *Drugs and Therapy Perspectives*, **8(7)**, 5–9.

Anon. (1996). What scope is there for improving the cost effectiveness of NSAIDs? *Drugs & Therapy Perspectives*, **8(9)**, 12–16.

Committee on the Safety of Medicines (CSM). (1994). *Relative safety of oral non-aspirin NSAIDs: Current Problems in Pharmacovigilance*. London: CSM/ Medicines Control Agency: 20.

Crosby, V., and Corcoran, R. (1996). Modes of administration of morphine in cancer pain. (Letter) *Br. Med. J.*, **313**, 687.

Daniels, L., Faull, C. and Blackshaw, C. The use of strong opioids for cancer pain in the community. *Br. J. Commun. Health. Nurs.*, **1(6)**, 328–334.

Deyo, R. (1996). Editorial: Acute low back pain - a new paradigm for management. *Br. Med. J.*, **313**, 1343–1344.

Doherty, M., and Jones, A.C. (1994). Osteoarthritis. *Med. Internat.*, **22(4)**, 129–136.

Doyle, D., Hanks, G., and MacDonald, N. (1993). *Oxford Textbook of Palliative Medicine*. Oxford University Press: Chapter 4, Symptom Management.

Expert Working Group of the European Association for Palliative Care (1996). Morphine in cancer pain: modes of administration. *Br. Med. J.*, **312**, 823–826.

Fallon, M. and O'Neill, W. (1994). Cancer Pain. *The Practitioner*, **238**, 101–107.

Finlay, I. and Forbes, K. (1994). Symptom control in palliative care. *UPDATE*, **48(3)**, 179–188.

Foley, K. (1995). Editorial: Pain relief into practice: Rhetoric without reform. *J. Clin. Oncol.*, **13(9)**, 2149–2151.

Frew, A.J., (1994). Non-steroidal anti-inflammatory drugs and asthma. *Prescribers' Journal*, **34(2)**, 74–77.

Kurowska, A., and Tookman, A. (1996). Morphine: yesterday's drug or yardstick for the future? *Br. J. Hosp. Med.*, **56**, 256–259.

MeReC Bulletin – National Prescribing Centre., (1996). Pain control in palliative care. July. Vol.7: 25–28.

O'Neill, W.M. (1993). Pain in malignant disease. *Prescribers' Journal*, **33(6)**, 250–258.

Royal College of Physicians. Guidelines for the diagnosis, investigation and management of osteoarthritis of the hip and knee. *J. R. Coll. Phys. Lond.*, **27(4)**, 391–396.

Vickers, A. (1996). Complementary therapies in palliative care. *Eur. J. Palliat. Care.*, **3(4)**, 150–153.

Multiple choice questions (MCQs)

(The following four statements are each followed by five answers. Please indicate whether each is true or false.)

1. **The following are true statements:**

   a) Aspirin is associated with Reye's syndrome.
   b) Ibuprofen may be given to children as well as adults.
   c) Phenylbutazone should only be used in the treatment of ankylosing spondylitis.
   d) Piroxicam and diclofenac can be given as once-daily preparations.
   e) NSAIDs are contraindicated in patients with peptic ulceration.

2. **The following statements about fentanyl are true:**

   a) Transdermal fentanyl allows constant delivery over 72 hours.
   b) One 25 ug per hour fentanyl patch gives pain relief over 24 hours equivalent to 90 mg of morphine.
   c) Fentanyl patches should not be applied repeatedly to the same area of skin.
   d) Fentanyl is a controlled drug only if administered transdermally.
   e) If fentanyl is administered transdermally its analgesic effect will be apparent within 1 hour.

3. **The following are true statements:**

   a) Dihydrocodeine is a controlled drug only if given by injection.
   b) Diamorphine is less soluble than morphine.
   c) Dextropropoxyphene is given in conjunction with paracetamol as co-proxamol.
   d) On its own dextropropoxyphene is a powerful analgesic.
   e) Unlike morphine, buprenorphine is non-addictive.

Answers on page 38

4. **The following are true statements:**

    a) Meptazinol is long-acting with a powerful analgesic effect greater than 12 hours.
    b) Unlike buprenorphine, nefopam is highly addictive.
    c) Carbamazepine can be used to treat trigeminal neuralgia
    d) Amitriptyline can be used in the treatment of post-herpetic neuralgia.
    e) Dextromoramide is less sedating than morphine, but has a short duration of action.

    Answers overleaf

MCQ answers

(A maximum total of 20 marks are available.)

1. T,T,T,T,T.
2. T,T,T,F,F.
3. T,F,T,F,F.
4. F,F,T,T,T.

3
Lowering blood pressure

Hypertension is a particularly common problem in primary care and its detection and treatment have considerable implications for the morbidity and mortality of the population. This is because of the clear association between uncontrolled hypertension and coronary events, heart failure and stroke.

Hypertension should be regarded as a disease rather than an illness because patients do not usually feel ill on presentation: it is often discovered by chance when screening those who attend with an unrelated problem. The dilemma faced by the doctor managing a patient with hypertension centres around deciding when drug treatment is justified. One must be confident that the long-term benefits of blood pressure reduction outweigh the inconvenience of taking regular treatment and any short-term discomfort. When patients first start to take drug treatment they may feel less well as they adapt to having a lower blood pressure and to any unwanted effects of treatment. The dilemma is most acute in elderly patients, for whom the benefits may be more immediate but who are least tolerant of over-treatment.

Management must always include non-pharmacological measures. For some patients, lifestyle changes, such as losing weight and increasing exercise, may be all that is required to control blood pressure. Because all drugs can cause unwanted effects, drug treatment should be reserved for patients with continuing and sustained hypertension which puts them at increased cardiovascular risk, and for those who have clearly not responded to non-pharmacological measures alone. Whatever management plan is agreed, the importance of good control must be emphasized and good compliance is vital.

Modified essay question (MEQ)

(The instructions for the MEQ appear in the manual on page xi.)

Peter is a 40-year-old accountant who is married with three children. He attends the well man clinic at your surgery, having not seen you for five years. His only past medical history of note is an appendicectomy when he was aged 20 years. The nurse who takes his blood pressure finds it to be 180/100 mmHg and gets the same reading after 10 minutes.

1.   What further information might you require?

2.   What is your plan of action?

You see Peter two weeks later at your surgery after one further reading of 180/100 mmHg. Your initial assessment revealed that there is no family history of hypertension or premature cardiovascular disease, but he drinks 30 units of alcohol per week and smokes 20 cigarettes a day. He takes no regular exercise, but does not add salt to his food. There were no abnormal physical signs apart from raised blood pressure and excess body weight for his height; his Body Mass Index (BMI) is 28 kg/m^2 (recommended range 20 to 25.)

3.   What is your plan of action now?

After three months his blood pressure remains at 180/100 mmHg. He has been unable to make any changes in his lifestyle and his weight is unchanged. All investigations are normal, including urine analysis, routine blood tests, ECG and chest x-ray.

4.   What is your plan of action now and why?

5.   What drug therapies are available?

Peter is very stressed at work, seems to be tense when he comes to see you and admits to being on edge all the time. His resting pulse rate in the surgery is 96/min.

6.   What drug might you consider prescribing and why?

7.   *You decide on a beta-blocker. Are there any absolute contra-indications to this therapy and what possible side-effects might Peter experience?*

8.   *What advice would you give Peter about stopping his therapy should he find the side-effects intolerable?*

Peter experiences no side-effects and his blood pressure remains well controlled on a beta-blocker. However, he comes to see you nearly 15 years later because he is now suffering symptoms of prostatism. He has read in a national newspaper that one particular group of anti-hypertensive drugs is beneficial in this area and may help the blood lipid profile.

9. *Which group of anti-hypertensives is he referring to?*

10. *Why would you caution him against changing agents?*

MEQ answers

(Numbers in brackets refer to the marks you would receive in the MRCGP examination for each part of the answer you mention. Please total your own score to provide self-assessment.)

1. Weight, height and body mass index (BMI) (1).
    Previous blood pressure readings, if any (1). Family history (1).
    History of stress (1). Smoking and alcohol history (2).
    Exercise history (1). Diet (1) – salt intake (1).
    Examination (1): cardiovascular system including – resting pulse (1); auscultation of carotid and renal arteries for bruits (1); fundoscopy (1).
    Urine analysis (1).

Comment

A family history of raised blood pressure is common in patients with essential hypertension, but lifestyle is also an important determinant of blood pressure. Body weight and its distribution, physical activity, and consumption of alcohol and salt are key factors.

Blood pressure is directly related to body weight or body mass index.[1] Apart from age, no other measured characteristic correlates more strongly or more consistently. The relation is particularly strong in individuals with central or upper body obesity. The reason is not entirely clear but probably involves insulin resistance.[2]

Regular alcohol consumption has a pressor effect in both normotensive and hypertensive individuals. The relation between dose and effect is linear when daily intake lies between one and seven units, and is common to all alcoholic beverages.[3]

Blood pressure is related to the daily intake of sodium salt but the effect is small when corrected for body weight and alcohol intake. Nevertheless, a proportion of hypertensive patients, especially older ones, show increased sensitivity to salt and may respond to sodium restriction.[4] Also anti-hypertensive agents will be more effective if the patient is not salt loaded.

Whereas stress affects blood pressure acutely, there is little evidence that it has an important effect on resting blood pressure in patients who are accustomed to its measurement, and stress management is ineffective.[5] However, the acute effects of stress and inability to relax can easily elevate blood pressure so that readings taken by a doctor or nurse may be appreciably higher than those measured by the patient himself (white coat hypertension). If such anxiety is suspected in a patient, twenty-four hour ambulatory blood pressure monitoring may be helpful to confirm or refute the diagnosis of hypertension.

Smoking a cigarette can cause brief elevation of blood pressure, but regular smoking has no sustained effect. However, smoking is more important than hypertension as a cardiovascular risk factor, and the combined effects of smoking and hypertension are more than additive.

Active and fit individuals appear to have lower average blood pressure readings than the physically inactive.

2.   To repeat his blood pressure on two further occasions (2) and review him if it is still raised (1).

Comment

Guidelines issued by the British Hypertension Society recommend that blood pressure be measured on at least four separate occasions before making a decision about drug treatment. On each occasion, blood pressure should be recorded at least twice, to the nearest 2 mm Hg, with the patient seated, using a conventional mercury sphygmomanometer and a cuff with an appropriate bladder size (the bladder should embrace at least 75% of the arm circumference). In mild hypertensives (diastolic BP 90–99 mmHg) and older patients with isolated systolic hypertension (systolic BP > 160 mmHg), with no organ damage, the period of assessment should be 3–6 months, during which non-pharmacological measures may be used to lower blood pressure.[6]

3.   **Advice**
     Lifestyle (1) e.g., exercise.
     Dietary (1) – reduce fat intake.
     Advise him to lose weight (1) and explain how (1).
     Reduce alcohol intake to no more than 2 units daily (1).
     Emphasise that blood pressure reduction is necessary to prevent against heart attacks and strokes (2).
     Leave advice regarding smoking cessation to a future consultation (1).
     Further investigations:
     Urine analysis to exclude glycosuria (1) & proteinuria (1).
     Urea and electrolytes (1).
     Random cholesterol (1).
     ECG (1).

Chest x-ray (1) if heart is enlarged clinically (or if size cannot be assessed clinically), or if warranted by additional respiratory symptoms (1).

Organize an appointment for review (1).

Comment

Weight reduction lowers blood pressure, and the effect is enhanced by sodium restriction, where appropriate. Reducing energy intake to achieve target body weight will also correct insulin resistance and lessen, or even eliminate, the need for anti-hypertensive drugs.[1] However, effective management requires specific advice on how to modify the diet, what foods to avoid, and recommendations about quantity.

The effect of alcohol on blood pressure is greater in obese and older people, and reducing daily consumption to one or two units lowers blood pressure to an extent similar to that achieved by weight reduction. Abstinence does not improve response and deprives patients of the beneficial effects of low dose alcohol on other cardiovascular risk factors, such as HDL cholesterol and inhibitors of thrombosis.[3]

Whereas acute exercise increases blood pressure to an extent determined by individual fitness and the level of exertion, regular isotonic exercise, such as running, cycling or swimming, at least three times a week for at least one month, lowers blood pressure and the effect is sustained for as long as training continues. In addition, energetic activity, such as brisk walking, heavy housework and digging in the garden, can be just as beneficial as a structured exercise programme provided it is regular and continuous for at least twenty minutes at a time. However, the effect of regular exercise is more predictable in obese patients than in non-obese, and should not be relied upon to reduce blood pressure; for safety's sake it is best deferred until blood pressure has been controlled by other measures.[1]

If the prospect of lowering blood pressure by lifestyle modification alone is good, it is reasonable to defer advice about stopping smoking until a future consultation. Although smoking is a more important cardiovascular risk factor than hypertension, it is extremely difficult to stop smoking and lose weight at the same time; successful weight reduction will lower blood pressure and boost morale, which may make it easier to stop smoking in due course. Nevertheless, a serious attempt to stop smoking should not be put off for more than a few months after presentation.

Investigation at this stage should be limited to the assessment of other cardiovascular risk factors (glycosuria, hypercholesterolaemia), and detection of organ damage or strain caused by raised blood pressure (urea and electrolytes, proteinuria, ECG, chest x-ray).

4. Consider drug therapy (1).
    Explain to the patient that therapy is necessary to prevent against heart attacks and strokes (2).
    Re-emphasize the importance of altering lifestyle (1).

Comment

The decision to add drug treatment to the management plan should not depend on blood pressure readings alone. Other cardiovascular risk factors, such as age, gender, family history, personal history of cardiovascular disease, diabetes, smoking and cholesterol, should also be considered, as should the presence of left ventricular hypertrophy or of end-organ damage, such as renal disease.[7]

The most explicit recommendations, from New Zealand, suggest that patients with blood pressure readings of 150–170 mm Hg systolic or 90–100 mm Hg diastolic should not be considered for drug treatment unless their risk of acquiring cardiovascular disease over the next ten years is at least 20%.[8]

5. **Drug therapies available are:**
    Thiazide diuretic (1)
    Beta-blocker (1)
    Calcium channel blocker (1)
    ACE-inhibitor (1)
    Directly acting vasodilator (hydralazine) (1)
    Centrally acting antihypertensive (1)
    Alpha-blocker (1)
    Angiotensin II receptor blocker (1)

Comment

The list of available therapies is deliberately comprehensive, although one would not consider using either a directly-acting vasodilator or a centrally-acting anti-hypertensive as a first-line agent. Selection depends on the individual patient and any contraindications to the use of particular alternatives. For example, one would be inclined not to select a thiazide diuretic for a patient with diabetes or gout, or a beta-blocker for someone with heart failure or asthma.

If there are no specific indications or contraindications, one should bear in mind that beta-blockers and thiazides are the only drugs that have been shown to reduce the risk of stroke; beta-blockers have cardioprotective effects (at least after myocardial infarction); and both these agents are very much cheaper than newer drugs (an important consideration when one is embarking on life-long therapy).[9] There is no evidence that the adverse metabolic effects of thiazides, which are unimpressive when using modern low dose regimens, compromise their beneficial effects. Nevertheless, it has been suggested that a beta-blocker should be preferred as first choice for younger patients and a thiazide for older ones (who tend to be less responsive to beta-blockers).[7]

6.   A beta-blocker (1), e.g., atenolol 50 mg once daily.
     It can reduce the somatic manifestations of anxiety (1) as well as blood pressure (1) and will slow the pulse rate (1).

7.   Absolute contraindication is asthma (2).
     Possible side-effects are: tiredness/lethargy (1); cold extremities (1); hypotension (1); impotence (1); sleep disturbance (1).

Comment

Fatigue and lethargy are common (22%) and dose-related, although many patients come to tolerate these symptoms after continued treatment. Hypotension should not occur if the dose is correct. Impotence and sleep disturbance are uncommon and unpredictable.

8.   Stopping a beta-blocker suddenly may precipitate pre-existing symptoms of anxiety with palpitations (1). You should therefore counsel the patient appropriately (1).

Comment

Abrupt discontinuation of a beta-blocker after long term treatment seldom causes serious problems except in patients with pre-existing ischaemic heart disease, in whom it can exacerbate angina and lead to sudden death. Nevertheless, long term treatment does reduce sensitivity to beta agonists and can result in rebound supersensitivity for up to a week following withdrawal. This is prevented if withdrawal occurs over a few weeks.

9.   Alpha-adrenoceptor blocking drugs (2).

Comment

Alpha-blockers antagonize the contraction of prostatic smooth muscle and decrease bladder resistance to urinary outflow. They may therefore be useful in the management of benign prostatic hyperplasia.[10] However, drug treatment should not be prescribed for men with lower urinary tract symptoms before seeking objective evidence of bladder outlet obstruction.[11]

10.   Why change if his blood pressure is well controlled with a beta-blocker? (1) Beta-blockers have a useful cardio-protective effect (1). An alpha-blocker can be used in conjunction with a beta-blocker (1).
      After such a long period of time his beta-blocker should not be stopped suddenly (1). Alpha-blockade can cause postural hypotension (1). Alpha-blockers should be introduced with caution to avoid first dose hypotension (1). The benefits of alpha-blockers with regard to prostatism may not be dramatic (1).

(Total possible marks = 66.)

References

1.   Alderman, M.H. (1994). Hypertension octet. Non-pharmacological treatment of hypertension. *Lancet*, **344**, 307–311.
2.   Williams, B. (1994). Hypertension octet. Insulin resistance: the shape of things to come. *Lancet*, **344**, 521–524.
3.   Kaplan, N.M. (1995). Alcohol and hypertension. *Lancet*, **345**, 1588–1589.
4.   Bennet, N.E. (1994). Hypertension octet. Hypertension in the elderly. *Lancet*, **344**, 447–449.
5.   Johnston, D.W. *et al.* (1993). Effect of stress management on blood pressure in mild hypertension. *Br. Med. J.*, **306**, 963–966.
6.   Petrie, J.C., O'Brien, E.T., Littler, W.A., de Swiet M. (1986). Recommendations on blood pressure measurement. *Br. Med. J.*, **293**, 611–615.
7.   Swales, J.D. (1994). Hypertension octet. Pharmacological treatment of hypertension. *Lancet*, **344**, 380–385.
8.   Jackson, R. *et al.* Management of raised blood pressure in New Zealand: a discussion document. *Br. Med. J.*, **307**, 107–110.

9. Sever, P. *et al.* (1993). Management guidelines in essential hypertension: report of the British Hypertension Society. *Br. Med. J.*, **306**, 983–987.
10. Oesterling, J.E. (1995). Benign prostatic hypertrophy. *N. Engl. J. Med.*, **332**, 99–109.
11. Abrams, P. (1995). Managing lower urinary tract symptoms in older men. *Br. Med. J.*, **310**, 1113–1117.

Multiple choice questions (MCQs)

(The following four statements are each followed by five answers. Please indicate whether each is true or false.)

1. ACE-Inhibitors:

a) Are sometimes associated with a persistent dry cough.
b) May relieve symptoms in patients who also have heart failure.
c) Do not compromise renal function if introduced gradually.
d) Are not recommended in patients with diabetes.
e) Are contraindicated in patients with bilateral renal artery stenosis.

2. Thiazide diuretics are:

a) First line therapy in newly diagnosed diabetics.
b) Recommended in patients who also suffer with gout.
c) Useful where the patient also has heart failure.
d) Neutral in their effects on blood lipids.
e) Commonly associated with hypokalaemia.

3. Methyldopa:

a) Can cause drowsiness.
b) Does not exacerbate asthma.
c) Can be used safely during pregnancy.
d) Can induce acute porphyria.
e) Produces a positive direct Coombs test in up to 90% of patients.

4. Calcium-channel blockers:

a) Are useful in patients who also have heart failure.
b) Are useful in patients who also suffer with angina.
c) Can cause ankle swelling (in the absence of heart failure) that should respond to treatment with diuretics.
d) Are associated with headaches and flushing.
e) Such as nifedipine, but not verapamil or diltiazem, interact adversely with beta-blockers.

Answers overleaf

MCQ answers

(A maximum total of 20 marks are available.)

1. T,T,F,F,T.
2. F,F,T,F,F.
3. T,T,T,T,F.
4. F,T,F,T,F.

Managing ischaemic heart disease

Ischaemic heart disease accounts for one in every five deaths in the United Kingdom and causes considerable morbidity. The last ten years have seen many advances in investigative techniques and drug therapies, in particular the use of lipid-lowering drugs to prevent ischaemic heart disease.

The GP's role in preventive health care is expanding rapidly and patients are keen for health checks. A patient attending a well person clinic will be asked about family history and other risk factors relevant to ischaemic heart disease. Many patients have their fasting lipids assayed and receive advice on the strength of the results. Such advice may not involve a prescription, since the need for drug therapy in patients with hyperlipidaemia depends on their absolute risk of coronary heart disease. This will be determined by other risk factors as well as serum cholesterol, such as smoking and coexistent conditions, such as diabetes and hypertension.

Patients at greatest risk are those with established ischaemic heart disease and those with a strong family history. This chapter focuses on a patient with angina and explores two dilemmas: when and how should preventive anti-anginal therapy be considered; and when should lipid-lowering drugs be introduced? The practicalities of managing an acute myocardial infarction occurring at home are also considered.

Modified essay question (MEQ)

(The instructions for the MEQ appear in the manual on page xi.)

George is a 55-year-old man who consults you about retrosternal discomfort whenever he has walked briskly during the last 6 weeks. It lasts for about 2 to 3 minutes and passes off quickly with rest. The discomfort does not radiate into his arms, but he likens it to a heavy weight on his chest. Yesterday evening, after eating a large meal from the local fish and chip shop, the symptom recurred and lasted about two minutes. George is not a man you see often, but judging by his nicotine-stained fingers he is a heavy smoker. He is 12 kg (2 stone) overweight for his height and you learn that his father died suddenly at the age of 42 with a heart attack.

1. Describe your management plan for George.

George returns to see you one week later. He has had daily retrosternal discomfort that has been relieved almost instantly by sublingual glyceryl trinitrate (GTN). The results of his investigations reveal that the total cholesterol concentration is 8.6 mmol/L. He has received his hospital appointment which is for four weeks hence.

2. What advice might you give George? Assuming that he is normotensive and there is no abnormality in his urine, what dilemmas do you face regarding his management? Is there any further information that you require?

George attends the hospital 4 weeks later, by which time his angina has become more frequent but is still relieved by GTN. During an exercise test at the hospital angina was manifest after minimal exertion. The letter from the hospital doctor asks you to start regular therapy for his angina while he waits for investigation with coronary angiography, and, as his cholesterol remains high at 8.9 mmol/L, to commence lipid-lowering therapy.

3. *Describe the different possible therapies (excluding surgery) that could be used to treat his angina and any disadvantages that they may have, and identify any dilemmas that you may face when selecting an appropriate therapy.*

4. *Dietary modification has not led to a reduction in his cholesterol since you measured it four weeks ago. The fasting*

lipid profile revealed HDL cholesterol 0.8 mmol/L, LDL cholesterol 6.1 mmol/L and triglycerides 4.4 mmol/L. Would you consider drug treatment at this stage, and if so, what? What precautions might you take in monitoring for any possible side effects?

5.   *Would you take any action regarding the rest of George's family. If so, what?*

George has been given drug treatment and his fasting cholesterol four months later is 5.5 mmol/L. You don't see him for a further two months until your receptionist interrupts during a busy morning surgery, in which you are running 30 minutes behind with your appointments. She tells you that George's wife is on the 'phone asking to speak to you as he has chest pain and keeps vomiting. You speak to her and the history is of severe left-sided chest pain which has come on suddenly; she says George is lying on the settee and is looking very pale. The family live six miles away from your surgery.

6.   *What is your initial management plan and why?*

On arrival at the house there is no sign of an ambulance and you enter the house to find the patient vomiting and holding his chest. As he is vomiting it is not possible to administer aspirin. Examination reveals a pale and distressed patient, with no cyanosis, a blood pressure of 110/75 mmHg and an irregular pulse of 80. Auscultating the chest suggests that the irregularity of the pulse is due to ectopic heart beats. The lung fields are clear.

7.   *What should you do next prior to the arrival of the paramedics? (You do not have an ECG machine.)*

Two weeks later George's son, who is now aged 25 years, consults you with a history of non-specific stabbing left-sided chest pains two or three times day for the last week which are a few seconds in duration. He thinks the pain makes him slightly breathless at the time and he is worried it might be his heart. This is understandable in view his father's recent heart attack.

8. *What is the likely diagnosis and your management plan?*

MEQ answers

(Numbers in brackets refer to the marks you would receive in the MRCGP examination for each part of the answer you mention. Please total your own score to provide self-assessment.)

1. Perform a thorough physical examination (1), including measurement of blood pressure (1), auscultation of the heart (1), and abdominal examination to exclude an obvious aortic aneurysm (1).
    Test urine for the presence of glucose (1).
    Arrange blood tests to check full blood count, renal function, fasting blood glucose and lipids (4). Consider checking thyroid function if there is any clinical evidence of thyroid disease (1).
    Perform an ECG to exclude a recent myocardial infarction, and to identify evidence of myocardial ischaemia, an indication of higher risk (1).
    Explain that you think he may have angina and tell him what angina is (2).
    Advise a smoking cessation programme (1) and modification of his diet (1).
    Suggest that he takes aspirin 75 mg daily (1).
    Give him a supply of glyceryl trinitrate (GTN) tablets and ask him to take one when he next gets an episode of retrosternal discomfort to ascertain its effect and so assist the diagnosis (2).
    Suggest referral for an exercise test, either directly or indirectly via a specialist (2).
    Arrange to review him in one week to discuss his results (1), and to ascertain the effect of GTN if he has required this (1).

2. Re-emphasise that he is to stop smoking (1).
    Recommend a weight-reducing diet as he is overweight anyway (1), but also to give him advice about eating less saturated fat (1), and relatively more carbohydrate (1), mono-unsaturated and poly-unsaturated fats (2).
        George has two problems: stable angina and a raised cholesterol. This presents you with two therapeutic dilemmas (1). First, does he need therapy to prevent angina and, if so, should this be initiated straightaway or should you wait until his hospital appointment in four weeks time? (2) Second, does he need therapy to lower his cholesterol or should he be given a trial of diet first? (2).

With regard to lipid-lowering therapy, you will require further information regarding his lipids (1). You know his total cholesterol, but not his HDL cholesterol, LDL cholesterol or triglyceride concentrations (3). A profile of his fasting lipids will help you to decide which lipid-lowering therapy might be helpful, assuming you feel that he should be treated straight-away rather than being given a trial of diet (1).

Comment

All patients having angina more than twice a week should be offered a regular anti-anginal agent. There is no reason to wait for specialist advice unless there is genuine uncertainty about the suitability of a particular patient for specific drugs.

Therapy with a lipid-lowering drug should never be introduced on the strength of a single measurement of serum cholesterol. Although dietary modification alone seldom reverses hypercholes-terolaemia, it can lead to worthwhile reduction in cholesterol concentration in some patients, and this, in combination with other lifestyle alterations, can substantially reduce cardiovascular risk. Stressing the importance of diet at this stage also prepares the ground for later introduction of drug treatment, with which dietary measures should always be combined.

Nevertheless, in someone who appears already to have coronary artery disease, one would not normally persist with diet alone for more than three months.

3. **There are four types of drug treatment to consider:**
    (a) beta-blockers: these are most useful in patients with angina of effort. The British National Formulary includes ten that are licensed for this indication; all are equally effective after dose titration but some must be taken in modified-release form to allow a dose interval greater than 8 hours, which increases their cost (3). Beta-blockers cause tiredness and coldness of the extremities (2). They depress myocardial function and this can lead to heart failure if left ventricular function is already impaired (1). All beta-blockers, even those that are selective for beta1-receptors, can precipitate bronchospasm in susceptible patients (1). They may impair glucose tolerance in diabetics and interfere with autonomic and metabolic responses to hypo-glycaemia (2). Sudden withdrawal of a beta-blocker can exacer-bate angina (and can precipitate a myocardial infarction) if no other anti-anginal therapy is being taken (2).

(b) long-acting nitrates: oral formulations include isosorbide dinitrate (ISDN) and its active metabolite, isosorbide mononitrate (ISMN), both of which are available in conventional and modified-release forms, and modified-release GTN (oral or buccal). GTN is also available in transdermal form (4). Nitrates cause headache, flushing and postural hypotension, which are dose-related (3). Regular uninterrupted dosing can lead to tolerance which compromises benefit, unless the regimen used allows blood nitrate concentration to fall to a low level for at least 8 hours in each 24 (2).

(c) calcium channel blockers: these fall into two groups: dihydropyridines (e.g. nifedipine, amlodipine) and others (diltiazem, verapamil) (2). All are effective in angina of effort (or at rest), although verapamil or diltiazem are usually preferred in patients who do not respond to, or are intolerant of beta-blockers (1). Dihydropyridines cause flushing, headache and ankle swelling (which does not respond to diuretics), whereas verapamil causes constipation (3). Verapamil and diltiazem can cause symptomatic bradycardia and precipitate heart failure if left ventricular function is already impaired (1). Like beta-blockers, sudden withdrawal of calcium channel blockers can exacerbate angina (1).

(d) nicorandil: this is a potassium channel activator with additional nitrate-like actions, which relaxes both arterial and venous smooth muscle (1). It appears to be as effective as alternative anti-anginal agents, but not more so (1). It may be useful in patients who are intolerant of alternatives but its value in combination therapy is not yet clear (1). Like dihydropyridines, it causes headaches and flushing (1).

Aspirin also has a role in angina, not in relieving symptoms but rather in reducing the complications of ischaemic heart disease; it should be introduced as soon as the diagnosis has been made, provided there is no absolute contraindication (2).

Each of the four types of anti-anginal agent is equally effective (1). Choosing the best drug for the individual patient depends on what coexisting conditions the patient has, and often involves deciding which drug will cause the least unacceptable unwanted effects (1). George has responded well to symptomatic use of nitrate and would probably tolerate regular nitrate well (1). Given that his symptoms are effort induced, allowing the blood nitrate concentration to fall overnight should not present a problem. Whereas a beta-blocker could prove the best choice for his angina of effort, as an overweight smoker he might be more aware of the fatigue associated with beta-blockers and more susceptible to their bronchoconstrictor effect (2). Calcium channel blockers would have no clear advantages or disadvantages, but are generally more expensive than nitrates or beta-blockers and cheaper than nicorandil (2).

Comment

Beta-blockers are most effective if daily dosage is adjusted to prevent the heart rate exceeding 100/min during moderate exertion. Although they are reputed to aggravate the symptoms of peripheral vascular disease, the evidence that they do so is inconclusive; a cardioselective agent should be preferred and claudication distance in the individual patient should be measured before and after starting treatment. The consequences of stopping beta-blockers are seldom serious if exercise is avoided for 24 hours after withdrawal but most authorities recommend gradual reduction of dosage over several weeks unless an alternative anti-anginal agent is substituted.

Whereas use of ISMN formulations involves fewer daily doses than use of ISDN formulations, they are no more effective after dose titration and significantly more expensive. Transdermal GTN is the most expensive of all nitrate formulations, but may be useful in patients with nocturnal angina, where the effect of a bedtime oral dose is insufficiently sustained. Tolerance can usually be avoided by eccentric dosing to ensure that when using ISDN in a thrice daily regimen the last dose of the day is taken at 6.00 pm, and that when using ISMN in a twice daily regimen the daytime dose interval does not exceed 7 hours. Formulations of ISMN that can be given once daily (e.g., Imdur) do not appear to lead to nitrate tolerance.

Calcium channel blockers are distinguished pharmacologically by their preferential effects in three tissues: the myocardium (verapamil > diltiazem > nifedipine), the cardiac conducting system (V > D > N), and vascular smooth muscle (N > D > V). Concern has been expressed recently that use of shorter acting dihydropyridines, such as nifedipine in its immediate release formulation, in patients with angina or hypertension may be associated with higher mortality. The published evidence is inconclusive but the consensus at present recommends preferential use of formulations that avoid high peaks of drug concentration, such as the modified-release forms of nifedipine or the more slowly eliminated amlodipine. This has the added advantage that treatment can be given in no more than two daily doses.

In patients who require combination therapy for angina, additive unwanted effects are best avoided by using a beta-blocker with either a nitrate or a dihydropyridine, or verapamil/diltiazem with a nitrate. There is no virtue in combining two drugs of the same class, and little evidence that using any three drugs together affords greater benefit than two.

4.   There are five types of drug treatment worth considering:

   (a) statins: (e.g., simvastatin, pravastatin) are highly effective in reducing LDL cholesterol (1), but have minimal effect on HDL cholesterol and modest effect on triglycerides (1). Prior to initiation of (and during) therapy liver function tests should be assayed because of the unwanted effects statins can have on liver enzymes (1).

   (b) anion-exchange resins: (e.g.,cholestyramine, colestipol) (1). These reduce LDL cholesterol, but have little effect on HDL cholesterol and aggravate hypertriglyceridaemia (2). They should be taken with water, an hour before, or four hours after, any other drugs to reduce possible interference with absorption (1).

   (c) fibrates: (e.g., bezafibrate, gemfibrozil) act mainly to reduce triglycerides (1), but also reduce LDL cholesterol and increase HDL cholesterol (1). Their disadvantages are that they can cause a myositis-like syndrome and can predispose to gall stones. (2).

   (d) nicotinic acid: reduces LDL cholesterol, increases HDL cholesterol and reduces triglycerides (3). However, side-effects, such as flushing, may be a particular problem (1).

   (e) fish oils (omega 3-marine triglycerides): are useful in the treatment of raised triglycerides, but may raise the concentration of cholesterol. (2).

   After 4 weeks treatment lipids should be assayed again to see if the treatment being used is beneficial. If response is unsatisfactory, dosage should be increased, according to the manufacturer's recommendations, and titrated against response. Sometimes a combination of drugs has to be given to achieve an optimal result.

Comment

In a man aged 55 years with angina and a serum cholesterol of at least 7.3 mmol/L the absolute risk of myocardial infarction and death is substantial even before allowing for the effect of smoking. One can expect significant benefit from lipid-lowering therapy, which should certainly prove cost effective. Statins inhibit the enzyme 3-hydroxy 3-methoxy glutaryl coenzyme A (HMG Co A) reductase, which controls the rate of cholesterol synthesis in the liver. They are contraindicated in patients with active liver disease or those who have persistent elevation of serum transaminases. The risk of muscle damage is greater in patients with renal impairment or hypothyroidism.

Fibrates activate lipoprotein lipase and reduce peripheral fat breakdown. Their use in combination with statins should be reserved for resistant cases as both can damage muscle tissue and enhance each others' effects in this respect.

Anion-exchange resins act by binding bile salts, thereby preventing their reabsorption. This enhances hepatic conversion of cholesterol to bile acids; as a result there is an increase in LDL-receptor activity and increased breakdown of LDL cholesterol.

Nicotinic acid inhibits production of lipoproteins by the liver. It has a useful additive effect when a statin or a fibrate fails to restore the lipid profile to normal. It is available only in 50 mg tablets, which is very inconvenient when the effective lipid-lowering dose can be as high as 2 g thrice daily. The inevitable flushing that occurs soon after each dose is prostaglandin-mediated and can be prevented by giving aspirin 75 mg 30 minutes beforehand.

Omega 3-marine triglycerides should be reserved for patients with severe isolated hypertriglyceridaemia.

The aim of lipid-lowering therapy in patients with established ischaemic heart disease is reduction of LDL cholesterol below 3.3 mmol/L. The dose of drug treatment should be titrated upwards every 6–8 weeks until this target has been achieved. If it has not been achieved after 6 months the patient should be referred to a specialist in lipid therapy.

5. Active steps should be made to invite other members of his immediate family who are aged 18 years or over for a health check (2) which includes fasting lipids and blood pressure measurement (2). Also, the opportunity should be used to advise on weight, smoking cessation, exercise and eating a healthy diet (4).

6. The patient is most likely suffering an acute myocardial infarction (1). An ambulance with paramedics should be summoned (1) and the patient also visited immediately by the GP (1). Ask your receptionist(s) to explain and apologize to waiting patients

that you have been called out on an emergency and that appointments may be considerably delayed.

Comment

In patients with suspected myocardial infarction, speedy transfer to hospital is essential. Thrombolytic therapy with streptokinase reduces mortality by 50% if given within the first hour, but the benefit dwindles with every hour that passes. The shorter the 'pain-to-needle' time, the better the chance of survival.

7. Insert an intravenous cannula in case intravenous medication is required (1).
   Administer intravenously an injection of morphine or diamorphine in combination with an anti-emetic (2) (e.g., Cyclimorph, which contains morphine tartrate 15 mg and cyclizine tartrate 50 mg in a 1 ml ampoule). (Or intramuscularly if appropriate resuscitation equipment is not readily available.)
   Reassure the patient as appropriate as he will be very distressed (1).
   Continue to monitor the clinical condition until the paramedics arrive.

Comment

Aspirin 300 mg (the tablet to be chewed, macerated and swallowed) is the best immediate treatment if a myocardial infarction is suspected in a patient who is not already taking low dose aspirin, provided the oral route is available. Morphine 15 mg (in one ampoule of Cyclimorph) is not an excessive dose for an overweight man but, in view of his smoking history, his respiratory effort should be watched carefully after dosing, especially if this was intravenous.

8. Many expressions can be used all signifying pain that is likely to be musculo-skeletal in origin (e.g., Tietze's syndrome, psychosomatic pain, costochondral pain) (2).

   Management should include:
   A careful physical examination (1) which, if normal, will itself be reassuring (1).
   An ECG to exclude any abnormality (1) and again to reassure (1).

Assuming there is no abnormality, to reassure and discuss whether some of his symptoms may be a reaction to his father's recent heart attack (2).

Suggest simple analgesia, such as paracetamol, if the problem persists (1).

Suggest that he makes a further appointment if the problem persists or worsens (1).

(Total possible marks = 121.)

Further reading

Anon. (1996). Management of hyperlipidaemia. *Drug. Ther. Bull.* **34**, 89–93.

Anon. (1996). Which drug for stable angina? *Drugs & Therapy Perspectives*, **8(6)**, 5–8.

Cowan, J.C. (1996). Prescribing nitrates in angina pectoris. *Prescribers' Journal*, **36(3)**, 130–34.

Dargie, H.J. (1996). Calcium channel blockers and the clinician. *Lancet*, **348**, 488–489.

McMurray J. and Rankin, A. (1994). Cardiology 1: Treatment of myocardial infarction, unstable angina, and angina pectoris. *Br. Med. J.*, **309**, 1343–1350.

North of England Stable Angina Guideline Development Group. (1996). North of England evidence based guidelines development project: summary version of evidence cased guideline for the primary care management of stable angina. *Br. Med. J.*, **312**, 827–832.

Pharaoh, P.D.P, and Hollingworth, W. (1996). Cost effectiveness of lowering cholesterol concentration with statins in patients with and without pre-existing coronary heart disease: life table method applied to health authority population. *Br. Med. J.*, **312**, 1443–1448.

Multiple choice questions (MCQs)

(The following four statements are each followed by five answers. Please indicate whether each is true or false.)

1. The following are true of the use of nitrates:

    a) The effect of glyceryl trinitrate lasts only 20 to 30 minutes.
    b) Glyceryl trinitrate can be used to dilate the cervix to aid IUD insertion.
    c) Isosorbide mononitrate is more effective than isosorbide dinitrate.
    d) Nitrates can cause flushing and headaches.
    e) Patients on long acting nitrates can develop tolerance.

2. The following are true of calcium channel blockers:

    a) They can cause flushing and headaches.
    b) They are useful in treating angina when heart failure is present.
    c) Amlodipine and nifedipine can be used to treat angina and hypertension.
    d) They do not reduce the risk of myocardial infarction in unstable angina.
    e) They can cause ankle swelling.

3. The following are true of lipid-lowering therapies:

    a) Liver function should be checked prior to starting a statin.
    b) The use of fibrates are associated with a myositis-like syndrome.
    c) Fish oils have little place in the treatment of hypertriglyceridaemia.
    d) Nicotinic acid is of value in lowering lipids due to its lack of side-effects.
    e) Anion exchange resins are more cost effective than statins for hypercholesterolaemia.

Answers on page 72

4. The following are true of beta-blockers:

a) Beta-blockers reduce the recurrence rate of myocardial infarction.

b) Beta-blockers are contraindicated in patients with intermittent claudication.

c) Sudden withdrawal of a beta-blocker can cause an exacerbation of angina.

d) Beta-blockers can impair glucose tolerance.

e) Beta-blockers can precipitate heart failure.

Answers overleaf

MCQ answers

(A maximum total of 20 marks are available)

1. T,T,F,T,T.
2. T,F,T,T,T.
3. T,T,F,F,F.
4. T,F,T,T,T.

5

Wheezing and dyspnoea

Wheeze and asthma are common problems for the general practitioner in patients of all ages. There appears to have been a worldwide increase in the prevalence of asthma, particularly in childhood. But the aetiology of the disease remains varied and controversial. There is also no clear-cut definition of asthma, particularly in children under age 5; doctors disagree on whether all children who have an episode of wheeze should be labelled as suffering with asthma. For these reasons the decision to treat and the choice of treatment vary among practitioners. There is concern about the unwanted effects of prophylactic inhaled steroids.

The timing, choice and intensity of treatment used for patients with asthma vary widely, and not simply because of difficulties with the diagnosis. Even when the diagnosis has been made, doctors vary in their willingness to prescribe inhaled corticosteroids, especially in children due to concern over unwanted effects, and to use oral corticosteroids for acute attacks. When symptoms become worse an antibiotic is often the first choice of treatment, partly in deference to patient (or parental) expectations; yet the guidelines drawn up by the British Thoracic Society make no mention of antibiotic therapy at any stage in the management of asthma.

The outcome of treatment for patients with asthma depends on the skill of the supervising clinician and the intensity of the monitoring and supervision offered. Good patient education is vital, especially in childhood and adolescence, to ensure proper understanding of how the treatment works and how it should be used, and to foster good compliance.

Dilemmas also arise in older patients (aged over 45), in whom the differentiation of asthma and chronic pulmonary obstructive disease (COPD) is often difficult. These patients are often treated as though they had asthma, on few clinical grounds, with little attention being paid to their underlying pathology.

Modified essay question (MEQ)

(The instructions for the MEQ appear in the manual on page xi)

John is aged 24 years and consults his GP having had a head cold for 3 days, a dry cough and unaccustomed shortness of breath on exertion. He is a known asthmatic, having suffered with seasonal asthma in the summer months since childhood, but has never required hospital treatment or oral steroids. He is taking inhaled salbutamol as required and beclomethasone 100 microgram inhaler two puffs twice daily. He is compliant with his treatment and attends the asthma clinic at the surgery regularly. On examination he is apyrexial and has no obvious abnormality of his throat, but has a few small lymph glands in his neck and the occasional expiratory wheeze in his chest. His peak expiratory flow (PEF) is 400 L/min with a predicted value of 550 L/min.

1.   What is your management plan?

John consults 2 days later and is having difficulty breathing while dressing and climbing stairs. His peak flow has dropped to less than 65% of his predicted value (350 L/min). On examination he is distressed with a temperature of 38°C, and rhonchi in both lung fields but no signs to suggest pneumonia. He is not cyanosed and his pulse is 88/min. He also tells you that he is now coughing up green sputum. You decide to give him nebulized salbutamol 5 mg in 2.5 ml of saline. Following this he feels much better and his peak flow returns to 480 L/min.

2.   What is your management plan now?

John comes to see you 2 days later and is having great difficulty breathing. His PEF has dropped to 55% of the predicted value (300 L/min). Your practice nurse has given him nebulized salbutamol 5 mg in 2.5 ml of saline and his peak flow changes to 320 L/min. You learn that he has only taken 10 mg daily of prednisolone and not the dose you recommended because he has 'heard worrying things' about steroids. He is leaning forward with his hands on his knees and cannot complete sentences without pausing to draw breath.

3.   Describe your management plan now.

One month later John comes to the surgery having recovered from his acute attack of asthma and is stabilized on beclomethasone 250 microgram inhaler 2 puffs twice daily. He has not come in to consult about himself, but about his 2-year-old daughter, Zoe. He wonders if Zoe might have asthma as she has been suffering with a persistent cough for the last 6 weeks. She had been brought to see your partner 2 weeks earlier, when she was given a course of antibiotics for a suspected chest infection, but there has been no improvement in her cough. On examination there is no abnormality of the ears, nose or throat. The lungs are clear and heart sounds normal. She is playing happily in a corner with some toys while you ask her father a few more questions.

4.   *What other information might you request from her father in an attempt to verify or exclude a possible diagnosis of asthma?*

5.   *You satisfy yourself that Zoe does not have an obvious upper respiratory tract infection (URTI) and is otherwise well. What might your management plan be?*

Some weeks later you are called to see a 60-year-old man at home who has just moved into the area. He gives a history of what sounds like wheezy bronchitis. He gives a long history of wheezing and uses a salbutamol inhaler regularly (2 puffs 4 times daily) and beclomethasone 250 microgram inhaler 2 puffs twice daily. Talking to him at length it transpires that he is John's grandfather, who has moved into the area to be near his family. He has been a heavy smoker for many years and continues to smoke 5 cigarettes per day; he says he cannot stop smoking and the cigarettes are the only thing that help 'bring the phlegm up'. He says his previous GP had requested a chest x-ray and told him that he had got emphysema. On further enquiry he has difficulty getting out of the house as a result of severe dyspnoea, but there is no history of an acute infection and his breathing has been like this for many months. On examination there is no evidence of heart failure and there are bilateral expiratory wheezes in both lung fields.

6.   *What is the likely diagnosis and how might you verify this?*

7.   *What treatment options could be considered for this patient?*

MEQ answers

(Numbers in brackets refer to the marks you would receive in the MRCGP examination for each part of the answer you mention. Please total your own score to provide self-assessment.)

1. Check his inhaler technique (1).
    Suggest that he doubles the dose of his inhaled beclomethasone while he is unwell (1).
    Suggest he uses his salbutamol as often as necessary (1).
    Advise him when he should reconsult, particularly if his PEF drops further, if he feels tight and his symptoms are not relieved by salbutamol for more than 2 hours, or if he has difficulty breathing at rest (3). Recommend also that he consult if he develops symptoms of a fever and shivering, which might imply the appearance of pneumonia (2), but emphasize the ineffectiveness of antibiotics in the routine management of asthma attacks (1). This information should be supplemented by a written personal plan detailing the thresholds for action and explicit guidance (2).

Comment

A routine check of inhaler technique, even in patients accustomed to using an inhaler, will often reveal imperfections that compromise the benefit of treatment. Even when technique is perfect, less than 10% of a metered dose of aerosol will be inhaled deep into the bronchial tree and remain adherent to the bronchial lining rather than being exhaled.

Patients with asthma whose PEF falls to between 65–80% of their best or predicted level may respond to a doubling of the daily dose of inhaled corticosteroid, thereby avoiding the need for prednisolone. However, any change will take 36–48 hours to become effective, so the sooner it is made the better. As PEF falls, patients feel the need to use their bronchodilator inhaler more often and they should be encouraged to do so, within defined limits. A steady fall in the dose interval signifies a reduction in responsiveness and should be interpreted as a warning that additional treatment is necessary to prevent the attack becoming severe. A high proportion of asthma deaths have occurred in patients who have relied on frequent doses of bronchodilator for too long before seeking medical help. Once the dose interval reaches 2 hours or the PEF falls below 65% of predicted or best, oral steroids should be introduced.

The routine use of antibiotics in patients with asthma who have no evidence of chronic obstructive pulmonary disease does not improve the outcome in an acute attack unless there is radiological evidence of pneumonia.[1,2] In general practice, a chest x-ray will not be immediately available and the doctor must rely on physical examination to determine which patients are at significant risk. Even where fever or purulent sputum signify an underlying bacterial infection, and often they do not, the temptation to prescribe an antibiotic should be resisted. The aim of treatment is to increase bronchial calibre, by reducing spasm and oedema, so that excess secretions can be expectorated; as with any infection confined within a lumen, 'drainage' alone is necessary.

2. Re-emphasize the ineffectiveness of antibiotics in this situation (1).
    Commence a course of prednisolone 30 mg daily for 10 days (1).
    Loan him a nebulizer to use 6 hourly if required (1).
    Review him daily until he is significantly improved (1).
    Review him immediately if he is worried or his peak flow drops further (1).

Comment

A short course of prednisolone will suffice to allow recovery. Provided that a daily dose of at least 30 mg is given for 10 days, prednisolone can be stopped without the need for tapered withdrawal in patients taking maintenance inhaled corticosteroid.[3] Inhaled steroid adds nothing to the effect of prednisolone, and could be withheld for most of the period of oral treatment to be reintroduced 48 hours before the oral steroid is withdrawn to ensure that there is overlap between the two. However, this complicates the instructions and risks inadvertent omission of inhaled steroid when oral treatment is withdrawn.

3. Order a 999 ambulance with paramedics to come to your surgery (1).
    Request that your practice nurse draws up 0.5 ml of 1:1000 adrenaline for injection should it be required (1).
    Ensure an airway is available if required and the necessary equipment to intubate (1).
    Insert an IV cannula (1).
    Inject hydrocortisone 200 mg IV (1).

If oxygen is available, give 40-60% by face mask (1).

Consider giving nebulized ipratropium bromide 500 microgram (2 ml of 0.025% solution). (1)

Do not leave John (1) and try to ensure he does not become excited (1).

Explain that as a precautionary measure you are going to ask a hospital doctor to see him and inform the resident medical officer at the local hospital that he is coming and needs to be seen straightaway (1).

Ensure the safe transfer of John to the local hospital and provide the receiving doctor with a letter detailing his history and medication (2).

Comment

Hydrocortisone will not be effective for 4 hours but its effect will appear sooner than that of an increased dose of prednisolone (6 hours). Nebulized ipratropium bromide and nebulized salbutamol (or terbutaline) have additive effects in acute severe asthma.[4] If ipratropium is not available, and the patient is not already taking either theophylline or aminophylline by mouth, one might consider giving aminophylline 5 mg/kg IV. However, this must be given by slow IV infusion over 20 minutes and should not be allowed to delay transfer to hospital. A high inspired concentration of oxygen (40%) is appropriate except in patients with evidence of chronic obstructive pulmonary disease, in whom a more modest concentration (24%) is preferable to minimize the risk of CO_2 retention.

4. **Questions that, if answered in the affirmative, might indicate asthma are:**

   Has there been a history of similar episodes in the past? (1).

   (How many courses of antibiotics has she had recently?)

   Is the cough mainly at night? (1).

   Apart from John does anyone else in the family suffer with asthma? (1).

   Is there a history of eczema? (1).

   Does either of Zoe's parents smoke? (1).

   Has John or his wife heard Zoe 'wheeze'? (1).

   Is the cough associated with exercise? (1).

   Was onset of cough related to the acquisition of a family pet? (1).

Questions that, if answered in the affirmative, might indicate a URTI are:
Is there a history of coryza? (1).
Is there purulent mucous discharge from her nose? (1).
Is there a history of fever? (1).
Has Zoe been unwell in herself or lethargic? (1).
Is Zoe off her food? (1).

5. Zoe is at a difficult age to use an inhaler or spacer device but a trial of bronchodilator therapy can be useful in the diagnosis of asthma. It might be appropriate therefore to suggest that Zoe is given 2.5 to 5 ml of salbutamol syrup (2 mg/5 ml) at night (assuming that her cough is worst at night) and to review her in a few days to see if there has been any response (2).
   If there is a good response to medication it would be appropriate to use a bronchodilator inhaler with a large volume spacer device such as salbutamol (Volumatic) or terbutaline (Nebuhaler) as required (2).
   If Zoe's symptoms are persistent and only partially relieved by the above medications one should recommend the additional use of sodium cromoglycate (5 mg metered dose from inhaler into large volume spacer device (Fisonair) 4 times daily) (1).
   If this approach is ineffective after 4–6 weeks, consider substitution of an inhaled corticosteroid for sodium cromoglycate (1).

Comment

Once the diagnosis of asthma has been made, the management plan should follow the guidelines recommended by the British Thoracic Society and endorsed by the British Paediatric Association. The aim of treatment is to abolish symptoms and allow the child to lead a full and active life. Symptoms should be monitored and written guidelines given to the parents.

The guidelines, which are less precise for children under 5 than for older children, suggest that treatment begins with 'as required' inhaled bronchodilator (using a large volume spacer), moving on to 'as required' inhaled bronchodilator with either regular inhaled sodium cromoglycate or inhaled corticosteroid (e.g., beclomethasone, budesonide, fluticasone). It is not clear which alternative would be more effective in a 2-year-old child, but sodium cromoglycate would probably prove more acceptable than inhaled corticosteroid to parents, in the first instance. If sodium cromoglycate remained ineffective after 4–6 weeks, an inhaled corticosteroid could be substituted with the confidence that it was now the only effective alternative. If symptoms persist after a further month, one should double the dose of the inhaled corticosteroid, and consider giving a 5 day course of oral corticosteroid (prednisolone). Older children may benefit from addition of a long-acting inhaled beta$_2$-agonist (e.g., salmeterol, which is licensed for use in children aged 4 years and over).

Ipratropium bromide is not superior to, and does not add useful benefit to, beta$_2$-agonists in the maintenance treatment of chronic asthma, but may be useful where beta$_2$-agonists are poorly tolerated. Sodium cromoglycate is more effective in children than in adults and should precede the introduction of corticosteroids, although growth retardation does not appear to be a significant problem with inhaled corticosteroids. Whereas fluticasone is twice as potent as either beclomethasone or budesonide (so that half the dose by weight achieves the same effect), the evidence that it is any safer than either beclomethasone or budesonide used with a spacer device is inconclusive; and once the daily maintenance dose of beclomethasone or budesonide reaches 800 micrograms, treatment should always be administered via a large volume spacer[5] (Volumatic or Nebuhaler, respectively). Portability is not an issue, even in older children, as the daily dosage of inhaled corticosteroid need not be divided into more than 2 doses.

6. It is likely that this is chronic obstructive airways disease (COAD), also called chronic obstructive pulmonary disease (COPD) (1).

    The diagnosis rests on:
    A long history of expectoration (1)
    A long history of smoking and a history of exercise limitation (2).
    A reduced PEF which does not vary during the day (1).
    A consistently reduced FEV$_1$, with FEV$_1$/FVC ratio < 75% (2) and poor reversibility of airways obstruction (< 200 ml or < 15% improvement in FEV$_1$ after nebulized bronchodilator) (2).
    A chest x-ray that shows hypertranslucent lung fields with no focal pathology (1).

7. **Short-term therapies:**
    Review inhaled medication and encourage compliance (2).
    Check inhaler technique (1).
    Commence a programme of smoking cessation (1).

Check that there is no infection (i.e., purulent sputum) requiring treatment with antibiotics (1).
Ensure a yearly influenza vaccination (1).

Long-term therapies:
Refer to physiotherapy for exercise and education (2).
Prompt treatment of acute infective episodes with antibiotics (1).
Use of beta$_2$-agonists for relief of symptoms (1). It may be necessary as the patient's respiratory function deteriorates to consider using these in a nebulizer (1).
Consider a trial of corticosteroids (1).
Consider modified release methylxanthines (aminophylline, theophylline). (1).
Oxygen for short-lived increases in breathlessness (1).

Comment

Of those patients with COPD whose airways obstruction is reversible, two therapeutic approaches are worth trying. Two-thirds will benefit from regular use of either a beta$_2$-agonist (e.g., salbutamol, terbutaline) or an anticholinergic (e.g., ipratropium bromide) inhaler; benefit from salbutamol/terbutaline in this patient group is often limited by unwanted effects, chiefly tremor. One-fifth will respond to corticosteroids, given initially as prednisolone 30 mg daily for a trial period of 14 days, with measurement of FEV_1 before and after to gauge response objectively. Those patients whose FEV_1 improves by $> 15\%$ and by > 200 ml should continue corticosteroid therapy, which is usually given in inhaled form. Those with severe disease ($FEV_1/FVC < 40\%$, disabling breathlessness and evidence of cor pulmonale) who do not respond to the above measures should be referred to a respiratory physician to consider whether long-term oxygen therapy (LTOT) should be prescribed. Controversy surrounds the use of inhaled corticosteroid in patients with COPD. Many respiratory physicians feel that the formal trial of oral steroids gives inconsistent results and favour the wider use of inhaled steroid. The outcome of clinical trials is awaited.

(Total possible marks = 71.)

References

1. Shapiro, G.G., Eggleston, P.A., Pierson, W.E., Ray, C.G., and Bierman C.W. (1974). Double-blind study of the effectiveness of a broad-spectrum antibiotic in status asthmaticus. *Pediatrics*, **53**, 867–872.
2. Graham, V.A.L., Knowles, G.K., Milton, A.F. and Davies, R.J. (1982). Routine antibiotics in hospital management of acute asthma. *Lancet*, **i**, 418–421.
3. O'Driscoll, B.R., Kalia, S., Wilson, M., Pickering, C.A.C., Carroll, K.B. and Woodcock, A.A. (1993). Double- blind trial of steroid tapering in acute asthma. *Lancet*, **341**, 324–327.
4. O'Driscoll, B.R., Horsley, M.G., Taylor, R.J., Chambers, D.K., and Bernstein, A. (1989). Nebulised salbutamol with and without ipratropium bromide in acute airflow obstruction. *Lancet*, **i**, 1418–1420.
5. Barry, P.W. and O'Callaghan, C. (1996). Inhalational drug delivery from seven different spacer devices. *Thorax*, **51**, 835–840.

Further reading

Anon. (1997). Using beta$_2$-stimulants in asthma. *Drug Ther. Bull.*, **35**, 1–4.

Barnes, P.J. (1995). Inhaled glucocorticoids for asthma. *N. Engl. J. Med.*, **332**, 868–875.

The British Guidelines on Asthma Management. (1997). *Thorax*, **52(2)**, Supplement S1–S21.

Jackson, C. and Lipworth, B. (1995). Optimizing inhaled drug delivery in patients with asthma. *Br. J. Gen. Pract.*, **45**, 683–687.

Keeley, D. and Rees, J. (1997). Editorial: New guidelines on Asthma Management. *Br. Med. J.*, **314**, 315–316.

Kolnaar, B. J. M. *et al.* Asthma in adolescents and young adults: screening outcome versus diagnosis in general practice. *Family Practice*, **11(2)**, 133–140.

Ninan, T. K., Macdonald, L. and Russell, G. (1995). Persistent nocturnal cough in childhood: a population based study. *Arch. Dis. Child.*, **73**, 403–407.

Rees, J. and Price, J. (1995). ABC of Asthma. Asthma in children: treatment. *Br. Med. J.*, **310**, 1522–1527.

Rees, J. and Price, J. (1995). ABC of Asthma. Treatment of chronic asthma. *Br. Med. J.*, **310**, 1459–1463.

Sibbald, B., Kerry, S., Strachan, D.P., and Anderson, H.R. (1994). Patient characteristics associated with the labelling of asthma. *Family Practice*, **11(2)**, 127–132.

Sturdy, P. *et al.* (1995). Characteristics of general practices that prescribe appropriately for asthma. *Br. Med. J.*, **311**, 1547–1548.

Weinberger, M, and Hendeles, L. (1996). Theophylline in asthma. *N. Engl. J. Med.*, **334**, 1380–1388.

Multiple choice questions (MCQs)

(The following four statements are each followed by five answers. Please indicate whether each is true or false.)

1. **The following steroid preparations are recommended in the prophylactic treatment of asthma:**

    a) Injection of Kenalog once every three months.
    b) Inhaled beclomethasone.
    c) Fludrocortisone 0.3 mg daily.
    d) Soluble Betnesol tablets in children.
    e) Inhaled budesonide.

2. **Drugs that may be used effectively in the treatment of acute asthma are:**

    a) Aminophylline.
    b) Salbutamol.
    c) Salmeterol.
    d) Oxprenolol.
    e) Terbutaline.

3. **Known side-effects of oral steroids are:**

    a) Osteoporosis.
    b) Disturbance of mental state.
    c) Muscle wasting.
    d) Acute gout.
    e) Peptic ulceration.

4. **The following drugs are suitable for inhalation in the treatment of asthma.**

    a) Salbutamol.
    b) Fluticasone.
    c) Aminophylline.
    d) Ipratropium bromide.
    e) Ephedrine hydrochloride.

Answers overleaf

MCQ answers

(A maximum total of 20 marks are available)

1. F,T,F,F,T.
2. T,T,F,F,T.
3. T,T,T,F,T.
4. T,T,F,T,F.

6

Type II Diabetes Mellitus

Type II diabetes, also known as non-insulin dependent diabetes (NIDDM) or maturity-onset diabetes, accounts for about 85% of all cases of diabetes in Northern Europe. It is common in middle-aged and elderly people (affecting 10% of people aged over 70 years) and its prevalence rises with age. A positive family history is the most important risk factor, but the condition tends to present when the genetically susceptible person develops obesity (particularly when this is abdominal). Hyperglycaemia results from both reduced insulin secretion (the mass of pancreatic beta-cells is reduced by about half) and reduced tissue sensitivity to insulin (insulin resistance).

Type II diabetes is usually of insidious onset with few or no symptoms; the classic symptoms of diabetes mellitus (polydipsia and polyuria) may not be present and are seldom dramatic. It is not unusual for the diagnosis to be made by chance during a routine medical examination. However, the condition reduces life expectancy in middle-aged patients by 5–10 years and should not be thought of as 'mild diabetes'. Like Type I diabetes (insulin-dependent diabetes; IDDM), Type II diabetes leads to vascular disease, which increases by two- to three-fold the risk of myocardial infarction and stroke, and damages the retina, kidney and peripheral nerves. Indeed, 10–20% of newly diagnosed patients with Type II diabetes already have significant arterial disease and retinopathy. Patients should be reviewed regularly to monitor the control of blood glucose and to identify and treat complications.

The most important aspect of treatment is diet. Although drug treatment is essential in Type I diabetes, it may not be necessary in Type II.

The greatest dilemma in the treatment of patients with diabetes is when to introduce treatment other than diet. This dilemma is accentuated when oral drug therapy fails to provide adequate control and a decision is required about when to introduce insulin therapy.

Modified essay question (MEQ)

(The instructions for the MEQ appear in the manual on page xi.)

Enid is a 55-year-old housewife and an infrequent attender at the surgery. Her main complaints are of tiredness and a small boil below her left axilla. Further questioning reveals that she has been tired for nearly a month, has become thirsty and has had considerable vaginal itching. She is 1.55 m tall and weighs 83 Kg (BMI = 35 kg/m^2). She smokes 10 cigarettes a day and drinks 10 units of alcohol per week. A random blood glucose is taken and the result is 20 mmol/L. You break the news to the patient that she has diabetes and she recalls that her mother had diabetes in later life.

1. *What would your management of the patient be?*

2. *You decide to recommend dietary advice in the first instance. What other parameters might you wish to measure that could have therapeutic implications for Enid?*

Enid is given a three-month trial on diet alone but her weight increases by 3 kg. She tests her blood each morning before breakfast and it usually indicates blood glucose between 12 and 15 mmol/L.

3.   What would be your management now and why?

4.   You decide to treat her with metformin 500 mg twice daily. What other drug treatments are available?

5. *The blood glucose concentration falls to normal over the next fortnight, but you find her to be hypertensive with an average blood pressure of 160/100 mmHg. What would be your first line anti-hypertensive and why?*

6. *The drug you prescribe produces an irritating and persistent dry cough and you decide to change her medication. What two groups of anti-hypertensives might you avoid and why?*

Enid responds well to metformin but over the next 4 years the dose has gradually to be increased to 850 mg tds; even this is insufficient to maintain control and you decide to start a sulphonylurea. You are telephoned by her husband during a busy morning surgery because she has not woken up. He has tried shaking her to no avail and wonders if she has had a stroke. You decide to visit immediately. There are no signs of a stroke and she has dilated pupils.

7. *What is the diagnosis and how would you manage her?*

8. *The diagnosis is hypoglycaemia. Is this an unwanted effect of all sulphonylureas? Is it more likely to occur with some agents than others and if so why?*

9. *Over the next 2 years she gains more weight and control of her diabetes is increasingly compromised. You detect microalbuminuria and fundoscopy reveals showers of hard exudates. Enid is now aged 61 years and has read about the serious effects that diabetes can have on the circulation, the kidneys and the eyesight. She asks whether these effects would be delayed more effectively if she used insulin. What are the pros and cons of insulin therapy in this patient?*

MEQ answers

(Numbers in brackets refer to the marks you would receive in the MRCGP examination for each part of the answer you mention. Please total your own score to provide self-assessment.)

1. She has probably had diabetes for several weeks and may be slightly dehydrated, which would account in part for the raised glucose concentration. You should encourage her to drink plenty of dilute sugar-free fluids (2), for example, carbonated mineral water which will also help to quench her thirst (1).

    Bearing in mind that she has just been given bad news, she will remember little of the consultation (1), particularly regarding lifestyle advice (1). Organize an appointment for review in a few days (2) and ask her to bring a list of questions (1) as there will undoubtedly be much that she wishes to ask about.

    Important lifestyle and dietary advice might include:
    Cut down on foods with a high sugar content, e.g., cakes and biscuits (2), and those with a high fat content (2).
    Aim to reduce weight and gradually to increase exercise (2).
    Try to avoid alcoholic drinks that have a high calorific value, e.g., beer and sweet wine (1). Stop smoking, to prevent this from accelerating the development of complications of diabetes (1). Emphasize that the mainstay of treatment is neither tablets nor insulin, but diet (2) and that this must be given as a trial for up to 3 months before considering the need for anything else (1).

Comment

This is not a medical emergency. Type II diabetes usually presents in this way and should be managed calmly, with the confident expectation that the blood glucose concentration will fall gradually over the next week or two and her symptoms will resolve. Educating the patient is the priority and this should be spread over several meetings to avoid information overload.

   Dietary guidelines suggested by the British Diabetic Association include:
Restrict daily calorie intake to 1000–1200 kcal, saturated fat to contribute less than 10% of total energy; increase mono- and poly-unsaturated fat so that total fat contributes up to 30% of total energy; carbohydrates, unrefined with a high fibre content, to con-

tribute 50% of total energy; protein to contribute 10–15% of total energy. Space meals evenly through the day and avoid snacks. List foods that should be avoided and those that are unrestricted. Prefer non-caloric sweeteners, such as saccharin and aspartame. Reducing body weight by 10–15% (8–12 kg in this case) would suffice to improve control of the blood glucose and reduce her body mass index to about $30 \, kg/m^2$. She should aim to stop gaining weight and try to achieve this target over 3–4 months. Emphasize that increased exercise is not merely desirable for good general health and to reduce the risk of heart disease, but is an important part of the treatment: exercise improves insulin sensitivity and contributes to lowering blood glucose and serum lipids. However, exercise cannot be relied upon to reduce body weight; only calorie restriction can bring this about.

2. Blood pressure (1) – is she hypertensive?
    Cholesterol (1).
    Test urine for protein: if absent then test for microalbuminuria (1), and arrange a blood test for creatinine (1) – what is her renal function like?

Comment

Hypertension is found in about 50% of newly diagnosed patients with Type II diabetes. Insulin resistance has been implicated in the pathogenesis of hypertension although the mechanism is not clear. Dyslipidaemia is also common and tends to be manifest as hyper-triglyceridaemia and reduced HDL cholesterol; total cholesterol concentration is commonly at the upper limit of the normal range, and LDL cholesterol is usually normal.

Microalbuminuria is characteristic of incipient diabetic nephropathy, the preclinical phase of overt diabetic nephropathy, which occurs in 10% of patients known to have had Type II diabetes for over 10 years. It is not apparent when the urine is tested with Albustix, but requires a more sensitive semiquantitative reagent strip and confirmation, if positive, by laboratory radioimmunoassay.

3. Ensure that she has seen a dietitian (1).
    Enquire about exercise (2).
    Encourage an increase in fibre intake (1).
    Consider drug therapy in addition to diet (1).

The first line drug therapy would be a biguanide – metformin, starting at a dose of 500 mg twice daily, increasing to a maximum of 850 mg 3 times daily (2).
She should be advised to take it after food to reduce the likelihood of gastrointestinal symptoms (1).

Comment

If diet and exercise, appropriately guided and supervised, have not achieved control of hyperglycaemia after 3–6 months, they are not likely to do so.
Biguanides reduce intestinal glucose absorption, stimulate anaerobic glycolysis and glucose uptake, and enhance insulin receptor binding and sensitivity; they do not affect insulin secretion and do not cause hypoglycaemia. However, metformin (the only biguanide licensed for use in the UK) causes gastrointestinal symptoms, such as anorexia, heartburn or diarrhoea, in 20–30% of patients.

4. A sulphonylurea (1), e.g., glibenclamide.
   Intestinal alpha-glucosidase inhibitor (1), e.g., acarbose. Guar gum (1). Insulin (1)

Comment

Sulphonylureas (e.g., chlorpropamide, glibenclamide, gliclazide, glipizide, tolbutamide) increase the sensitivity of pancreatic beta-cells to glucose and so promote insulin release. Their main unwanted effect is excessive hypoglycaemia, which is especially likely to occur in the elderly. A biguanide would be preferable to a sulphonylurea in an overweight patient because sulphonylureas, by increasing insulin secretion, stimulate appetite and are likely to cause even further weight gain.
Acarbose inhibits intestinal alpha-glucosidase, the enzyme that digests polysaccharides, and so reduces absorption of glucose. It causes flatulence, abdominal bloating and diarrhoea, especially during the first few weeks of treatment.
Guar is a soluble fibre extracted from the cluster bean, which impairs glucose absorption, possibly by affecting gut motility. Granules are sprinkled on the food. Guar can also cause troublesome gastrointestinal symptoms.

5. An angiotensin converting enzyme (ACE) inhibitor (1);

these drugs have been shown to reduce the progression of diabetic nephropathy (1), particularly in IDDM (1).

Comment

ACE inhibitors, unlike other anti-hypertensive drugs, have reno-protective effects that do not depend on their ability to lower blood pressure. In patients with microalbuminuria they postpone the development of macroproteinuria and of end-stage renal failure. Preliminary results suggest that these effects are not confined to patients with Type I diabetes, but also apply to those with Type II. ACE inhibitors should be introduced gradually, particularly in the elderly, as they can impair renal function and cause hyperkalaemia when there is unsuspected bilateral renal artery atheroma.

6. Thiazide diuretics (1), which can have an adverse effect on blood glucose and lipids (2), but this is generally minimal even in patients with diabetes (1).
    Beta-blockers (1), which theoretically can reduce glucose tolerance (1) and also interfere with the metabolic and autonomic response to hypoglycaemia (1).

7. Confirm that she is hypoglycaemic (1) with blood glucose test strips (1) and give her an intravenous injection of up to 50 ml of 50% glucose (1) assuming that it is not possible to give her sugar or glucose orally (1). If you are unable to find a vein for giving this infusion, give an intramuscular (IM) injection of glucagon 1 mg (1 unit) (1).

8. Yes – the effect is dose related (2), but the risk that hypoglycaemia will occur unpredictably (1), and not simply because a meal has been missed (1), is greater with compounds that have long elimination half-lives, e.g., chlorpropamide. Unexpected and prolonged hypoglycaemia is especially likely to occur when these drugs are used in elderly patients and in those whose renal function is impaired (plasma creatinine > 150 micromol/L). Glibenclamide may also cause this complication, chiefly because its active metabolites are excreted by the kidney. In patients with impaired renal function compounds with short elimination half-lives that have no active metabolites (e.g., tolbutamide, gliclazide) should be preferred (2).

9. **Pros**
   Improved control of her diabetes (1)
   A reduced rate of progression of complications (1)
   If blood glucose concentration is lower then she may feel better
   (1)
   A lower risk of intercurrent infection (1)
   Cons
   Adjusting lifestyle (1) and learning how to administer injections
   (1)
   Education of her family (1)
   Learning to monitor her blood glucose (1)
   Greater risk of hypoglycaemic episodes (1)
   Weight gain (1)
   Increased frequency of clinic reviews (1)

(Total possible marks = 67.)

Further reading

Anon. *Drugs & Therapy Perspectives.* (1996). Use ACE inhibitors for persistent microalbuminuria in diabetes. **7(11)**, 10–13.

Benn J.J., Sörksen P.H. *Med Internat.* (1993). Diabetes. **21(7)**, 237–282.

Gerich, J.E. (1998). Drug therapy: oral hypoglycaemic agents. *N. Engl. J. Med.*, **321**, 1231–1245.

Moller, D.E, and Flier, J.S. (1991). Insulin resistance – mechanisms, syndromes, and implications. *N. Engl. J. Med.*, **325**, 938–948.

Williams, G. (1994). Management of non-insulin-dependent diabetes mellitus. *Lancet*, **343**, 95–100.

Yki-Jarvinen, H. (1994). Pathogenesis of non-insulin-dependent diabetes mellitus. *Lancet*, **343**, 91–95.

Multiple choice questions (MCQs)

(The following four statements are each followed by five answers. Please indicate whether each is true or false.)

1. **The following statements are true:**

    a) Acarbose does not cause flatulence.
    b) Acarbose interferes with sucrose absorption.
    c) Diet alone can be an effective therapy in the treatment of diabetes.
    d) Guar gum needs to be taken with fluid.
    e) A glucose tolerance test (GTT) is necessary to make the diagnosis of diabetes.

2. **The following statements are also true:**

    a) A GTT involves an initial oral dose of 75 g of glucose.
    b) Guar gum should be taken last thing at night.
    c) Guar gum is unlikely to cause any gastrointestinal symptoms.
    d) Glucagon is a polypeptide hormone.
    e) Glucagon is produced by the beta cells of the Islets of Langerhans.

3. **Treatment with a sulphonylurea can cause:**

    a) Hypoglycaemia.
    b) Weight gain.
    c) Reduced beta-cell activity.
    d) Dangers to the baby if taken by a breast-feeding mother.
    e) Lactic acidosis.

4. **Treatment with a biguanide can cause:**

    a) Hypoglycaemia.
    b) Weight gain.
    c) Reduced beta-cell activity.
    d) Lactic acidosis.
    e) Constipation.

Answers overleaf

MCQ answers

(A maximum total of 20 marks are available)

1. F,T,T,T,F.
2. T,F,F,T,F.
3. T,T,F,T,F.
4. F,F,F,T,F.

7

Gastrointestinal disturbance

This is a particularly common aspect of practice and one in which therapies are advancing rapidly. There are two main therapeutic dilemmas. First, should one investigate every patient, or treat empirically and observe the response? Second, some symptoms are the result of inappropriate lifestyle, for example, where excess gastric acid is produced as a result of heavy smoking or where gastro-oesophageal reflux occurs in the overweight patient who continues to eat an unhealthy diet. It is easy for patients to become reliant on drugs that reduce or stop gastric acid secretion and prevent symptoms, when attention to lifestyle may not only avoid the need for drugs but would benefit general health. This has implications for drug budgets and general well being of patients.

Gastrointestinal disturbance is particularly common in children, both as a result of viral gastroenteritis and as a manifestation of other conditions, such as acute otitis media, where vomiting may be the predominant symptom. Also, where abdominal pain is recurrent in young children, urinary tract infection should be considered.

When referral is required there can be a management dilemma about whether to refer to a physician or a surgeon. Endoscopic techniques have revolutionized diagnosis and underpinned the choice of therapy, and can now avert the need for abdominal surgery in many situations. Similarly, laparoscopic surgery is useful both to make diagnoses and treat conditions such as gall stones.

Modified essay question (MEQ)

(The instructions for the MEQ appear in the manual on page xi.)

John is aged 21 and works as a local accountant's clerk. He comes to see you with a 2 month history of recurrent abdominal pain and what he describes as 'bloating'. He also describes intermittent episodes of alternating diarrhoea and constipation. On further questioning there is no loss of appetite and no rectal bleeding. However, you have seen him a couple of times in the last 6 months for insomnia that appeared to follow the sudden death of his father. During the consultation John seems very tense, but general and abdominal examination reveal no abnormality.

1. *What is the differential diagnosis and what therapeutic*
    possibilities might you suggest to John?

John is the oldest in his family and he has a younger brother, Dominic, aged 8. You are called out late one evening to see him because he has been crying with tummy ache for the last 4 hours. There is no history of diarrhoea or vomiting and he ate sausage and chips for his tea. Further questioning reveals that he has had a cold and a sore throat for the last 2 days. On examination there are a few tender and slightly swollen lymph glands in his neck and his throat appears red. Abdominal examination reveals a soft abdomen with minimal, but generalized tenderness and normal bowel sounds. He has a temperature of 37.5°C.

*2.   What is the most likely diagnosis and what treatment options
are available?*

Dominic's mother is aged 45 and comes to you a few weeks later.
She has been suffering for the last month with recurrent retrosternal
pain a short while after food, particularly when she bends over. She
has been understandably upset following the sudden death of her
husband and has been overeating. She is 1.6 m (5′ 3″) tall and
weighs almost 95 kg (15 stone). Examination is otherwise
unremarkable and she is a non-smoker.

*3.   What might be the problem and what therapeutic advice might
you give her?*

Unfortunately her symptoms persist and she comes 2 months later complaining of recurrent epigastric pain, which is waking her at night. Examination of the abdomen reveals epigastric tenderness and you find that she has lost 3 kg ($\frac{1}{2}$ stone) in weight. You suggest that hospital referral is necessary to exclude a gastric or duodenal ulcer. However, she is reluctant because her husband died in the hospital; she still has recurrent nightmares about his experience in coronary care where he arrested, was resuscitated, but arrested again fatally 2 days later.

4. *What therapeutic options might alleviate her symptoms? Why are you so keen for her to undergo further investigation?*

Fortunately, her symptoms resolve following a single 4 week course of cimetidine and she strives further to lose weight. However, John consults you again. He has been made redundant and his irritable bowel syndrome (IBS) has worsened. He is not sleeping and having weepy episodes. He tells you that he has had two episodes of fresh rectal bleeding when he has wiped his bottom after defaecation. Examination reveals no obvious abnormality of the abdomen, but two small haemorrhoids.

5. *What drug therapy is available to treat his haemorrhoids and what practical advice might you give him?*

John returns 2 months later with increasing abdominal pain, diarrhoea and tenesmus. The diarrhoea is occasionally bloody and he appears to have lost weight. Examination reveals mild tenderness in the left iliac fossa and rectal examination produces fresh blood on the glove. The ESR is raised at 50 mm in the first hour but the haemoglobin remains within normal limits and the albumin concentration is normal. You suggest referral to a hospital specialist, but again, for similar reasons to his mother, he refuses and is obviously petrified at the thought.

6. (a)   *What diagnoses might go through your mind?*

    (b)   *What appropriate investigations could you order at the surgery?*

(c)   What other investigations might be appropriate?

(d)   What information should be shared with the patient to ensure that he realizes the importance of attending a local hospital outpatient clinic?

MEQ answers

(Numbers in brackets refer to the marks you would receive in the MRCGP examination for each part of the answer you mention. Please total your own score to provide self-assessment.)

1. The most likely diagnosis is of irritable bowel syndrome (IBS) (1), but inflammatory bowel disease (1) or the possibility of a particular food intolerance (1) should be considered.

    Therapeutic options would be to explain what IBS is, that it is a common complaint and that it is not serious. Non-pharmacological methods might be suggested, such as increasing the amount of dietary fibre (1), taking regular exercise (1) and undertaking any activities that he enjoys and that enable him to relax (1). Suggest that medication can be used if symptoms become intolerable (1). Options include bulking agents, such as ispaghula husk (Fybogel Orange or Regulan) (1). Drugs, often referred to as antispasmodics (e.g., mebeverine), may also help (1). However, the problem is more ideally sorted out through appropriate dietary modification so that reliance on drugs does not ensue (1).

    Finally, if John's symptoms persist or do not settle, he should be advised to consult again in case he does indeed have inflammatory bowel disease (1) or an alternative diagnosis (1).

Comment

IBS has traditionally been thought of as a syndrome resulting from overactivity of colonic smooth muscle, but it can affect the whole gastrointestinal tract, sometimes presenting with non-ulcer dyspepsia. It is important to make a positive diagnosis and not to suggest or imply that the problem is wholly psychological. Investigation should be directed towards excluding other diagnostic possibilities suggested by symptoms that are not part of the IBS symptom complex, and kept to a minimum, especially in patients aged under 45 years. Treatment, which is largely empirical, comprises a bulking agent (where constipation predominates), an antispasmodic (for pain and bloating) and, if necessary, an anti-diarrhoeal preparation.

Ispaghula husk should be preferred to bran (especially wheat bran) which can make bloating and diarrhoea worse. Lactulose (an osmotic laxative) should be reserved for those in whom bulking agents are ineffective, though it, too, can make bloating worse. Another alternative, where constipation predominates, is cisapride, a prokinetic agent which acts on the myenteric plexus and increases small bowel and colonic transit. Certain antispasmodics, such as mebeverine, alverine and peppermint oil, have direct relaxant effects on smooth muscle, whereas others, such as dicyclomine and hyoscine butylbromide, have anticholinergic effects. They are all equally effective, usually within a few days, but individuals may respond better to one than to another. Unwanted effects are uncommon, but once symptoms are controlled an 'as required' regimen is recommended. Among anti-diarrhoeal preparations, loperamide is preferred to codeine phosphate, being less likely to cause dependence. Anti-depressants should usually be reserved for those with overt depression; anxiolytics have no place in patients with this disorder, but psychotherapy and hypnosis can be effective.

Although some rare diagnostic alternatives, such as laxative abuse, thyroid disease, or giardiasis can be excluded in general practice, patients who fail to respond to the above measures may need to be referred to a gastroenterologist for further investigation or 'specialist reassurance'.

2. The most likely diagnosis is of mesenteric adenitis (1). which is often associated with an upper respiratory infection. However, conditions such as 'abdominal migraine' (a precursor of adult migraine) and urinary tract infection should also be considered (1). Full advice should be given to his mother on when to consult again should his symptoms persist or increase in severity, just in case he is developing appendicitis (1).

    Three possible therapeutic options are available if you are confident that Dominic does not have appendicitis. First, to suggest he takes 500 mg of paracetamol in elixir or tablet form (1). Second, to consider antibiotic therapy (penicillin V) for his sore throat in the days to come should he develop signs suggestive of a bacterial tonsillitis (1). Third, to consider the use of antispasmodics if his abdominal symptoms persist, having satisfied yourself that examination excludes the likelihood of both appendicitis and other conditions, such as meningitis (2).

3. The most likely diagnosis is gastro-oesophageal reflux disease (1). You would advise her that she must lose weight (1) and purchase an over-the-counter antacid-alginate combination, such as Gaviscon, for symptomatic relief (1). This should also be taken regularly after meals and at night for one week or until her symptoms resolve (1). Dietary advice is also important, not

only to assist weight reduction; she should eat regular but small meals, and avoid spicy and fatty foods (2).

Comment

Gastro-oesophageal reflux disease (GORD) comprises a spectrum in respect of the degree of mucosal inflammation and the severity of symptoms. Reflux is often asymptomatic, and even among those with symptoms only a minority seek medical help. Heartburn and the sensation of gastric contents rising up the oesophagus are typical symptoms that often respond simply to an adjustment in lifestyle. Weight loss, reduction of alcohol intake and fatty foods, and the avoidance of large meals and bedtime snacks, may be all that is necessary, although some patients will need to elevate the bed head, to prevent night-time reflux, and stop smoking. For those who fail to respond or to comply with these measures, several medical treatment options are available: in less severe cases alginate-containing antacids (Gaviscon, Gastrocote) are often preferred, though standard antacids may be equally effective.

4. Antacids can again be tried (1) or an H_2 antagonist (1), such as cimetidine (1) or ranitidine (1). If symptoms persist despite 4 weeks treatment with an H_2 antagonist and she still declines investigation, you could try a proton pump inhibitor (1), such as omeprazole, or cisapride (1) which increases lower oesophageal pressure.

    You are keen to investigate because she may have an active ulcer or, at age 45, a neoplasm (2). Ulceration might also be due to infection with *Helicobacter pylori*, eradication of which requires triple therapy using a local treatment protocol (2). This could be detected using a serological test or a 'breath test' (2).

Comment

Where symptoms suggestive of GORD persist or worsen despite antacids and attempts to modify lifestyle, referral for endoscopy is advisable. Provided this does not reveal mucosal erosion, H_2 antagonists are often effective except in the most severe cases. Only where these are ineffective at standard dosage (e.g., cimetidine 400 mg twice daily, ranitidine 150 mg twice daily), or endoscopy reveals erosive oesophagitis, should a proton pump inhibitor (e.g., lansoprazole, omeprazole) or a prokinetic agent (e.g., cisapride) be considered. With modern medical treatment, surgery (fundoplication) is rarely necessary.

If endoscopy reveals peptic ulceration, the possibility of infection with *H. pylori* should always be considered. Among patients with duodenal ulcer, 95% are infected, and among those with gastric ulcer, 80%. If infection is confirmed by finding urease-producing organisms in the gastric antral biopsy, or using an isotope breath test, or by finding circulating antibodies to *H. pylori* in the serum, the infection should be eradicated. This not only heals the ulcer without the need for a lengthy course of treatment with an ulcer-healing agent, but greatly reduces the likelihood of recurrence after healing. Many authorities would now recommend 'blind' eradication therapy in all patients with duodenal ulcer, without confirmation of the presence of *H. pylori*.

There are numerous alternative antibacterial regimens. Most include one or two antimicrobial agents (e.g., amoxycillin, clarithromycin, tetracycline, metronidazole), with either bismuth chelate (a topical antimicrobial) or an acid suppressant (e.g., proton pump inhibitor, H_2 antagonist) to enhance the effect of the antimicrobials. Those comprising three agents are more effective than those comprising two, and more acceptable than those comprising four. Because of changing fashions in this treatment area, as well as changing resistance patterns, especially with respect to metronidazole, it is best to seek local gastroenterological advice regarding the currently preferred regimen. Although no regimen can claim 100% success, eradication is usually effective within 1–2 weeks and can be assumed if symptoms are relieved and do not recur; it need not be confirmed objectively except in patients who have experienced complications, such as bleeding. If confirmation is required, the breath test should be repeated at least 4 weeks after completion of treatment. Serological evidence of *H. pylori* will persist for at least a year after successful eradication.

5. Drug therapy includes the use of a stool softener (1), such as lactulose, and topical creams or suppositories containing local anaesthetic and steroid (cortisone.) (2). Practical tips that you can give him are to avoid straining at stool (1), not to ignore the call to defaecation (1), and to eat a high fibre diet (1). It may also be appropriate to discuss his father's death and to organise bereavement counselling if this seems appropriate (1). Anxiety will inevitably exacerbate his IBS symptoms.

6   (a)   **Inflammatory bowel disease**
          Ulcerative colitis (1).
          Crohn's colitis (1).
          Infective colitis
          Bacterial (e.g., Campylobacter, Salmonella) (2).
          Amoebic (1).
          Pseudomembranous (1).
    (b)   Stool culture (1).
          Repeat haemoglobin, ESR and albumin to monitor the
          condition (1).
    (c)   Proctoscopy (1).
          Sigmoidoscopy (1).
          Colonoscopy (1).
          Barium enema (1).
    (d)   A diagnosis needs to be made (1).
          If he has inflammatory bowel disease it may progress if it
          goes untreated (1).
          Colitis of more than 10 years duration is associated with an
          increased risk of bowel cancer (1), even in patients who
          have enjoyed lengthy remissions.
          It is possible to make him feel better and remove his symp-
          toms (1).

(Total marks available = 60.)

Further reading

Irritable Bowel Syndrome (IBS)

Farthing, M.J.G. (1995). Irritable bowel, irritable body, or irritable brain. *Br. Med.
J.*, **310**, 171–175.
Lynn, R.B. and Friedman L.S. (1993). Irritable bowel syndrome. *N. Engl. J. Med.*,
329, 1940–1945.
Weber, F.H. and McCallum, R.W. (1992). Clinical approaches to the irritable bowel
syndrome. *Lancet*, **340**, 1447–1452.
Whorwell, P.J. (1992). The irritable bowel syndrome. *Prescribers' Journal*, **32(4)**,
152–156.

Gastro-oesophageal Reflux Disease (GORD)

Colin-Jones, D.G. (1996). Gastro-oesophageal reflux disease. *Prescribers' Journal*,
36(2), 66–72.
Pope, C.E. (1994). Acid-reflux disorders. *N. Engl. J. Med.*, **331**, 656–660.

Helicobacter pylori

Dixon, M. (1993). Acid, ulcers, and H. pylori. *Lancet*, **342**, 384–385.

Phull, P.S., Hayward, P., Applethwaite, G., Everitt B. and David, A. (1996). Absence of dyspeptic symptoms as a test for *Helicobacter pylori* eradication. *Br. Med. J.*, **312**, 349–350.

Savarino, V. and Vigneri. S. (1995). How should we decide the best regimen for eradicating Helicobacter pylori? *Br. Med. J.* **311**, 581–582.

Walsh, J.H. and Peterson, W.L. (1995). Drug therapy: the treatment of *Helicobacter pylori* infection in the management of peptic ulcer disease. *N. Engl. J. Med.* **333**, 984–991.

Multiple choice questions (MCQs)

(The following four statements are each followed by five answers. Please indicate whether each is true or false.)

1. **Groups of drugs that may promote the healing of peptic ulcers include:**

   a) Antacids.
   b) H_2-receptor antagonists.
   c) Antimuscarinics.
   d) Liquorice derivatives.
   e) Aminosalicylates.

2. **Useful anti-diarrhoeal drugs include:**

   a) Paracetamol.
   b) Co-codamol.
   c) Loperamide.
   d) Domperidone.
   e) Peppermint oil.

3. **The following statements about constipation are true:**

   a) Constipation is related to the use of paracetamol.
   b) Constipation is a particular problem with NSAIDs.
   c) In the young, constipation is ideally treated using co-danthrusate.
   d) Faecal softeners, in particular, liquid paraffin, should be used first.
   e) Constipation responds well to domperidone.

4. **Irritable bowel syndrome may respond to:**

   a) Peppermint oil.
   b) Prochlorperazine.
   c) Ispaghula husk.
   d) Omeprazole.
   e) Domperidone.

   Answers overleaf

MCQ answers

(A maximum total of 20 marks are available)

1. T,T,T,T,F.
2. F,T,T,F,F.
3. F,F,F,F,F.
4. T,F,T,F,F.

8

Menstrual regulation and dysfunction

Throughout a woman's reproductive life malfunction of the reproductive organs, symptoms arising from their normal function, or a desire to interfere with their normal function, can present dilemmas for the doctor. For example, how far should one intervene to alleviate symptoms, such as painful menstruation, premenstrual tension, or age-related menstrual irregularity? Where does one's responsibility lie when asked to assist in the termination of a potential but unwanted pregnancy? To what extent is infertility a medical problem? How does one reconcile the benefits and risks of oral contraception, especially in the older woman, or of hormone replacement therapy as reproductive life draws to its close?

Some would argue that the individual woman should be free to order the function of her body as she chooses, enlisting medical assistance as and when required. Others would disagree, claiming that these are matters of moral and ethical significance, too important to be left to the individual. While this debate continues doctors (usually GPs) will face issues such as these in their everyday practice and be obliged to weigh in the balance the consequences and costs of intervention and non-intervention, treatment and non-treatment, when attempting to make the right decision.

Unfortunately, the hormone preparations discussed may have potential and as yet unknown long-term side-effects. Thus, with this concern in mind it is difficult to fully inform patients of all the possible risks of such therapies. This raises medico-legal implications and the use of a consent form may soon be appropriate.

Modified essay question (MEQ)

(The instructions for the MEQ appear in the manual on page xi.)

Sally is aged 16 years and has been having painful periods for the last 4 years following her menarche. She comes to the surgery alone and initially seeks advice concerning a sore throat.

1.   *Having excluded a throat problem, you make various*
     suggestions to treat her dysmenorrhoea. What might they be
     and in what circumstances would you feel that potential
     remedies were contraindicated?

Sally is prescribed a non-steroidal anti-inflammatory drug (NSAID) and consults you again after 3 months to request some emergency contraception. She is mid-cycle and has had unprotected intercourse on a single occasion 2 days earlier. Apparently she got drunk at a party and knows nothing of the person she had intercourse with. She is still suffering with dysmenorrhoea and asks your advice. Finally she tells you she has a boyfriend and she is keen that he does not find out.

2.   *What is your advice to Sally and what options are open to you?*
     Indicate the pros and cons of each option.

You decide to start Sally on a combined oral contraceptive pill (e.g., Microgynon 30). However, after 3 months she consults you with a history of repeated focal migraine and concern with regard to the amount of weight that she has put on since she started the 'pill'. She asks what alternatives are available for contraception. (She states that she would prefer not to use barrier methods because they are messy and she is worried about all the 'problems' associated with IUCDs.)

3.   Discuss the alternatives and their pros and cons.

Sally marries and has three children. She is now aged 43 and attends your surgery to inquire whether she is going through 'the change of life'. Direct questioning reveals that she has been suffering heavier and more painful periods for the last 6 months, and that the interval between her periods has dropped from 4 to 3 weeks and sometimes less. She also volunteers that she has been feeling more tired than usual, having the occasional night sweat and being tearful on many occasions without any obvious reason.

4. *What would you say to Sally and what therapeutic dilemmas does she present for you? What are your therapeutic options, bearing in mind that this is a very common problem in practice?*

Sally comes to see you 12 months later. She is now having periods every 2 weeks. They are very heavy (she is passing large clots) and they are lasting up to 7 days. Her haemoglobin is 8.3 g/dL with evidence of iron deficiency, she feels very tired and she is constantly tearful. She has been to a gynaecologist who has diagnosed moderately sized uterine fibroids and suggested that she may benefit from a hysterectomy. However, she is worried that if she has the operation that she may lose what she describes as her 'womanhood'.

5. *What would you say and what therapeutic interventions would you try to implement?*

Sally comes to you after 3 months. She has had no further periods and her latest hormone analysis indicates that she is menopausal. She is suffering with almost constant and disabling hot flushes and feeling depressed. She is accompanied by her husband who has already commented that your surgery is running late and is repeatedly fidgeting with his mobile phone. Sally becomes tearful and her husband says that she has become impossible to live with and they have not had sex for 9 months and that 'you must do something'. Sally asks, 'Would HRT help?'

6. *Outline the pros and cons of HRT to Sally and her husband.*

7. *What non-hormone therapies are available to treat menopausal symptoms?*

MEQ answers

(Numbers in brackets refer to the marks you would receive in the MRCGP examination for each part of the answer you mention. Please total your own score to provide self-assessment.)

1. The importance of keeping a menstrual diary (1) and enquiring what analgesic medication is presently being used (1). Mefenamic acid is the NSAID of choice for dysmenorrhoea as it reduces both pain and menstrual flow (1). However, caution should be exercised if there is a history of previous upper gastro-intestinal tract problems (1) or a history of asthma, particularly if associated with nasal polyps (1). The next possible option is prescription of the oral contraceptive pill in an attempt to regulate her periods (1), and to reduce pain (1) and menstrual flow (1). However, the prescription of this is contra-indicated if there is a history from the patient of arterial or venous thrombosis (1), severe hypertension (1), ischaemic heart disease (1), severe or multiple risk factors of arterial disease (1), liver disease (1), focal or severe migraine (1) or episodes of transient cerebral ischaemia (1). Additional contra-indications include a history of hydatidiform mole (1), cholestatic jaundice (1), deterioration of otosclerosis (1), breast or genital tract carcinoma (1), undiagnosed vaginal bleeding (1) and breast feeding (1).

Comment

Primary dysmenorrhoea, occurring in young women for the first few years after ovulation begins, results from an increase in prostaglandin and leukotriene synthesis consequent upon cyclical changes in oestrogen and progesterone concentration. The ensuing myometrial contraction and vasospasm lead to uterine ischaemia and pain. The most consistently reliable analgesic is a cyclo-oxygenase inhibitor. Whereas mefenamic acid was the first NSAID to be licensed for use in the treatment of dysmenorrhoea, there is no pharmacological reason to doubt that other related drugs (e.g., diflunisal, flurbiprofen, ibuprofen, ketoprofen, naproxen) are similarly effective; indeed, given the inter-individual variability in response to different NSAIDs in other painful conditions (e.g., inflammatory arthritis), it would be reasonable to try an alternative agent in this group if one's initial choice is not, or is only partially, effective.

Oral contraceptives are not intended to relieve but to prevent dysmenorrhoea, by suppressing ovulation and thus the normal cyclical changes in the balance between oestrogen and progesterone. Physiological menstruation does not occur and cyclical bleeding is seldom associated with more than trivial discomfort. Ninety per cent of young women with primary dysmenorrhoea obtain substantial relief from the introduction of an oral contraceptive and 50% obtain virtually complete symptomatic relief.

2.   Counsel the patient that pregnancy is unlikely, but possible (1). Discuss the following options and ask her to make a choice (1). a) The morning-after pill (1), alias the proprietary compound, Schering PC4 (1), involves taking 4 tablets, each of which contain 50 micrograms of ethinyloestradiol and 250 micrograms of levonorgestrel (3). If this is to be effective 2 tablets should be taken within 72 hours of sexual intercourse and 2 tablets 12 hours later (2). Give Sally full advice regarding symptoms of pregnancy and when to reconsult you if she is worried (1).

Pros
The simple regimen when taking the medication (1).

Cons
Its use is subject to the usual contraindications to the oral contraceptive pill (1).
It can cause nausea and vomiting (1); disturbance of menstrual cycle (1); headache (1); breast discomfort (1).

b) For post-coital contraception, an intrauterine contraceptive device (IUCD) can be inserted up to 120 hours (5 days) after intercourse (2).

Pros
Can be used up to 5 days after intercourse (1).
Highly effective – more so than the hormonal method (1).

Cons
Discomfort (1) and risks of insertion (1).
Introducing an infection into the uterus (1).
Difficulty of inserting an IUCD in a nulliparous woman (1).

Suggest future contraceptive options after the request for emergency contraception has been prescribed (1), including the oral contraceptive pill (2). Advise her to tell her parents (1).

Discuss future plans for contraception and when to consult if she is worried (2).

Comment

The recommended dose of Schering PC4 (4 tablets) is intended to prevent implantation of the fertilised ovum in the endometrium. It does not prevent ectopic implantation, so if pregnancy occurs despite its use (the failure rate is about 2%), tubal implantation should be carefully considered. The risk of teratogenesis is negligible, especially if the first dose is taken within 72 hours of coitus, and there is no need to consider therapeutic abortion. The efficacy of hormonal post-coital contraception may be impaired if the woman is already taking certain other drugs, such as phenobarbitone, phenytoin, rifampicin, griseofulvin, or broad-spectrum antibiotics.

Almost all combined oral contraceptives contain ethinyl oestradiol and one of six alternative progestogens. Once effective (immediately if started on day 1 of menstruation; within 7 days if started thereafter) ovulation is prevented and does not recur until contraception is withdrawn (deliberately or accidentally) for more than a week. In monophasic 'pills' the dose of the two components is fixed, whereas in biphasic and triphasic compounds the formulation varies during the monthly cycle in an attempt to mimic physiological fluctuations in sex hormone concentration. It is customary to start with a monophasic formulation, substituting an alternative only if persistent breakthrough bleeding occurs. Unwanted effects, such as irregular bleeding, breast tenderness and headache, usually disappear after the first two cycles; if they persist, substitution of a formulation containing a different progestogen may help. Pre-existing migraine is not an absolute contraindication unless associated with neurological signs, but the effects in the individual sufferer are unpredictable.

Newer progestogens (e.g., gestodene, desogestrel and norgestimate) are more selective and have lesser effects on serum lipids, carbohydrate metabolism and blood pressure. However, it is not clear whether these differences will result in clinical advantages, and against them must be set the higher incidence of venous thromboembolism now known to be associated with the use of gestodene and desogestrel. These progestogens therefore should no longer be regarded as first line treatment in these age groups, unless there are specific indications.

Combined oral contraceptives afford excellent protection against pregnancy and its associated risks, and have added advantages over non-hormonal methods, such as a reduced incidence of benign breast disease, cancer of the endometrium and ovary, dysmenorrhoea, menorrhagia, ovarian cysts and pelvic inflammatory disease. The risks include a dose-dependent increase in the incidence of venous thromboembolism and myocardial infarction, as well as a slightly increased incidence of carcinoma of the liver, breast and cervix.

3. The progesterone-only contraceptives can be considered, either in oral (1) or injectable form (1).
    Oral progestogen-only contraceptives. Several different preparations exist; their advantages include fewer side-effects than are associated with combined contraceptive pills (1), and the fact that they are taken every day so the patient does not have to remember to have a 7 day break (1). This group of drugs is suitable for breast-feeding mothers (1), and older patients who are hypertensive or who smoke (1). Their disadvantages include a possible risk of failure even if they are taken correctly (1); the fact that they have to be taken within 3 hours of the same time every day (1); their potential to cause menstrual irregularities (1); and less complete protection against ectopic pregnancy than against intrauterine pregnancy (1).
    Parenteral progestogen-only contraceptives. These are long-acting progestogens (1) that are as effective as combined oral preparations (1). These preparations are effective immediately (1), but they can cause menstrual disturbance (1), delayed return of fertility (1), or irregularity of periods after treatment has been discontinued (1). Depot preparations are most likely to result in amenorrhoea if used long term. Implant alternatives offer the almost immediate reversibility of their contraceptive effect (1).

Comment

Progestogen-only contraceptives render cervical mucus impenetrable to sperm, and the endometrium unsuitable for implantation; they also alter tubal motility and sometimes suppress ovulation. All contain non-selective progestogens, and the effects of an oral dose do not last longer than 24 hours. They do not increase the incidence of venous thromboembolism but are less effective than combined formulations when given by mouth, especially in young women.

4. First, explain that the 'change in life' or menopause is defined by cessation of menstruation (1) and thus reassure her that this is not the menopause yet, even though she may be approaching it (1). Explain in understandable terms that she is suffering with what appears to be menorrhagia and stress that this is a common experience prior to the menopause (2). Describe how her

symptoms may settle or may worsen (2). Finally, tell her that you may be able to offer her a greater prediction as to whether she is entering the menopause with a blood test to measure her hormone levels (FSH, LH, oestrogen and prolactin) (2).

Therapeutic dilemmas – should you:

(a) take the view that the symptoms are a physiological consequence of middle age that require no specific action? (1).

(b) entertain the possibility that there might be a pathological cause? (1).

(c) feel impelled to restore her menstrual cycle to 'normal' using any means at your disposal? (1).

(d) worry that increased blood loss might result in anaemia? (1).

Therapeutic options – do you:

(a) do nothing except reassure and plan to review? (1).

(b) perform a vaginal examination to exclude uterine fibroids or other pathology? (1).

(c) prescribe iron tablets? (1).

(d) assay haemoglobin and hormone levels and treat as appropriate? (2).

(e) suggest that she keeps a chart of her menstruation (1) and use a progestogen, such as norethisterone, cyclically? (1).

(f) refer her to a gynaecologist? (1)

5. State that a hysterectomy would help the present problem, but that it is a major operation (2). It would be wise to stay on the hospital waiting list for the operation in case the medication you are going to suggest does not work (2). Reassure her that her periods may stop if she does indeed go through the menopause (1). Ensure that she is given iron tablets (1) and that she is taking them (1). Suggest that she takes norethisterone 5 mg 3 times daily for 10 days to halt menstruation and then from days 5 to 25 of the menstrual cycle (3). Consider the use of other progestogens, e.g., dydrogesterone (1), or drugs that interfere with gonadotrophin release (e.g., danazol) (1).

Comment

Menorrhagia affects one in five women and involves excessive bleeding, passage of large clots, and social disability. All women presenting with these symptoms should have a pelvic examination and a full blood count. If, in addition, cycle length is altered or irregular, especially in a woman over 40, an endometrial biopsy should be requested (to exclude hyperplasia or malignancy) before assuming that the change is due simply to dysfunctional uterine bleeding, which should respond to medical management alone.

If there is no alteration in cycle length, or an endometrial biopsy is normal, the first choice of medical treatment is a cyclo-oxygenase inhibitor, such as mefenamic acid; other NSAIDs, such as diclofenac, ibuprofen or naproxen, are equally effective, but are not licensed for use in this way. If mefenamic acid is poorly tolerated, an alternative is ethamsylate, which probably acts by increasing platelet aggregation and capillary wall resistance. If anaemia has already occurred, tranexamic acid, which inhibits plasminogen activation and reduces the increased fibrinolytic activity in the endometrium during menstruation, should be preferred, together with ferrous sulphate. Tranexamic acid will reduce blood loss by half, but can cause nausea, vomiting and diarrhoea, and should be avoided if there is a history of thromboembolism.

A combined oral contraceptive, which is worth considering in a non-smoker, will reduce menstrual blood loss and regularize cycle length if menorrhagia is associated with an ovulatory cycle, whereas progestogen-only contraceptives, although they may prolong cycle length, will be much less effective. However, if cycles are anovulatory, a 10-day course of norethisterone will halt bleeding and subsequent cyclical use (days 5–25) will prevent recurrent excessive loss. Non-androgenic alternatives to norethisterone include dydrogesterone and medroxyprogesterone.

Other medical approaches involve interference with normal gonadotrophin release. Danazol, which suppresses gonadotrophin release and has a direct anti-oestrogenic effect on the endometrium, reduces menstrual blood loss but can cause undesirable alteration of cycle length, amenorrhoea or constant spotting, as well as weight gain, acne and deepening of the voice. It should not normally be continued beyond 3 months because of its androgenic effects on serum lipids. Gonadorelin (gonadotrophin-releasing hormone) analogues (buserelin, goserelin, leuprorelin, nafarelin) suppress ovulation and induce amenorrhoea. They will control severe menorrhagia but are not at present licensed for this use.

If medical management fails, or is contraindicated or poorly tolerated, hysterectomy, or the more recent technique of endometrial ablation, may be justified.

6. **Pros:**
   Provision of symptomatic relief (1).
   Reduce risk of the development of: osteoporosis (1), heart disease (1).

Cons:

Depending on the type of HRT chosen she may menstruate
again (1).

Increased risk of breast cancer after 5–10 years (1).

The need for regular health checks (1).

Comment

Hormone replacement therapy (HRT) is intended to make good the
deficiency of oestrogen that occurs after the menopause and to prevent its consequences, which can be immediate or delayed. The
immediate effects are vasomotor symptoms, such as attacks of flushing and sweating, and atrophy of the lower genital tract. The delayed
effects are more serious. The rate of bone demineralization after the
fourth decade is the same in men and women until periods cease,
after which time it doubles for 5–10 years before settling back to the
previous rate; half of all bone loss in women is attributable to the
menopause, and by age 70 half of all women will have had at least
one osteoporotic fracture. The risk of coronary artery disease,
against which premenopausal women are largely protected, increases
in postmenopausal women even more sharply than in men; compared with men, women who sustain a myocardial infarction are
more likely to die or, if they survive, to reinfarct, and the mortality
from coronary artery disease in postmenopausal women is 29%.

These consequences can all be influenced by oestrogen replacement. The immediate effects of the menopause are prevented, the
delayed effects attenuated. In the case of osteoporosis, oestrogen
replacement (opposed or unopposed by progestogen), given either
by mouth, transdermally or by subcutaneous implant, restores calcium balance and reduces bone turnover to its premenopausal level
for as long as treatment continues: treatment for as little as 5 years
reduces the risk of hip fracture by 50–75%, but the protective effect
wanes after withdrawal and is negligible by age 75. Where coronary
artery disease is concerned, the benefits are less certain; although
unopposed oral oestrogen replacement appeared to reduce the incidence of coronary disease by up to 45% in case-control and obser-
vational studies, selection bias (in favour of healthier women) may
have improved the outcome, as the incidence of cancer was also
reduced. Nevertheless, unopposed oestrogen replacement (by whatever route) corrects menopausal changes in serum cholesterol, and
opposed oral oestrogen replacement also improves the lipoprotein
profile, so there are grounds for optimism pending the outcome of
further trials.

Against these benefits must be set the risks. Unopposed oestrogen replacement increases the risk of endometrial cancer (fivefold after 5 years and more than tenfold after 10); the effect can be eliminated by taking progestogen for 12 days each month. Oestrogen replacement (opposed or unopposed) for 5 years increases the risk of breast cancer by 50% if given soon after the menopause, and by 70% if given to older women (age 60–64); it is not known whether the increased risk is sustained after replacement ceases. HRT is associated with a twofold to fourfold increase in the risk of venous thromboembolism but the increased risk appears to be restricted to the first year of use. However, the absolute risk remains low: no more than one or two additional cases of venous thromboembolism per 10 000 women per year would be expected. There is no evidence that HRT increases the incidence of cervical or ovarian cancer, nor that it has any adverse effects on hypertension or diabetes.

HRT with oestrogen and cyclical progestogen causes cyclical bleeding, at least initially, and this reduces its acceptability. There is therefore increasing interest in alternative forms of replacement that are less likely to have this effect. Tibolone, a synthetic compound with oestrogenic, progestogenic and androgenic effects, resolves menopausal symptoms and prevents bone demineralization but causes bleeding in only 15% of women; newer compounds combine oestrogen with continuous low dose progestogen (equivalent to 12 days cyclical therapy), which renders the uterus atrophic and leads to amenorrhoea in 95% of women after 12 months use. Because these compounds are given continuously, they should not be started until a year after the last natural period in order to avoid uncertainty about the nature of any postmenopausal bleeding.

7. **Hot flushes**
    Clonidine hydrochloride (50 micrograms twice daily) may be prescribed (1).
    Insomnia
    Non-addictive hypnotic preparations may be considered (1).
    Depression
    Antidepressants may be considered (1).
    Atrophic vaginitis
    Topical oestrogen cream (e.g., Ortho Dienoestrol 0.01% cream) may be considered for short-term use (1).
    General menopausal symptoms
    Pyridoxine (50 mg daily) may be helpful in some cases (1).

(Total available marks = 111.)

Further reading

Anon. (1995). Has HRT come of age? *Lancet*, **345**, 76–77.

Belchetz, P.E. (1994) Hormonal treatment of postmenopausal women. *N. Engl. J. Med.*, **330**, 1062–1071.

Davidson, N.E. (1995). Hormone-replacement therapy – breast versus heart versus bone. *N. Engl. J. Med.*, **332**, 1638–1639.

Jacobs, H.S. and Loeffler, F.E. (1992). Postmenopausal hormone replacement therapy. *Br. Med. J.* **305**, 1403–1408.

McPherson, K. (1995). Breast cancer and hormonal supplements in postmenopausal women. *Br. Med. J.*, **311**, 699–700.

Pérez Gutthann, S., García Rodriguez, L.A., Castellsague, J. and Duque Oliart, A. (1997). Hormone replacement therapy and risk of venous thromboembolism: population based case-control study. *Br. Med. J.*, **314**, 796–800.

Posthuma, W.F.M., Westendorp, R.G.J. and Vandenbroucke, J.P. (1994). Cardioprotective effect of hormone replacement therapy in postmenopausal women: is the evidence biased? *Br. Med. J.*, **308**, 1268–1269.

Prescribers' Journal, Symposium: Topics in gynaecology, **34(6)**, 205–242.

te Velde, E.R. and van Leusden, H.A.I.M. (1994). Hormonal treatment for the climacteric: alleviation of symptoms and prevention of postmenopausal disease. *Lancet*, **343**, 654–658.

Multiple choice questions (MCQs)

(The following four statements are each followed by five answers. Please indicate whether each is true or false.)

1. **The following measures will relieve or prevent dysmenorrhoea:**

   a) Combined oral contraceptive.
   b) Progestogen-only contraceptive.
   c) Ibuprofen.
   d) Paracetamol.
   e) Insertion of an IUCD.

2. **Dysfunctional uterine bleeding can be attenuated by treatment with:**

   a) Mefenamic acid.
   b) Tranexamic acid.
   c) Danazol.
   d) Combined oral contraceptive.
   e) Progestogen-only contraceptive.

3. **The following statements are true of combined oral contraceptives**

   a) They reduce the incidence of pelvic inflammatory disease.
   b) They are contraindicated in women with varicose veins.
   c) They are not contraindicated in women with migraine, provided there are no focal neurological signs.
   d) They should be withdrawn once women reach age 35 years.
   e) In women taking enzyme-inducing drugs (e.g., phenytoin, carbamazepine), a formulation containing at least 50 μg of ethinyl oestradiol and a monthly pill-free interval of 4 days are recommended.

4. **Hormone replacement therapy:**

   a) Is the most effective treatment available for relief of acute menopausal symptoms.
   b) Increases bone mineral content in postmenopausal women.
   c) Is as effective when given transdermally as it is by mouth.
   d) Is contraindicated in women with hypertension, even when blood pressure is controlled.
   e) Increases the incidence of breast cancer after treatment has continued for 5 years.

Answers overleaf

MCQ answers

(A maximum total of 20 marks are available)

1. T,F,T,T,F.
2. T,T,T,T,T.
3. T,F,F,F,T.
4. T,T,T,F,T.

9

Migraine

Migraine is a common disorder that can present a diagnostic and therapeutic conundrum for many sufferers and practitioners. To some extent this relates to the discrepancy between migraine as perceived and defined by medical practitioners, and the variety of symptoms their patients experience; and this may explain the frequent failure of conventional remedies.

Classic migraine begins with an aura, comprising symptoms such as loss of vision, awareness of flashing lights, tingling and numbness, or transient defects in speech or motor functions. These symptoms then subside and are followed by a severe throbbing headache, usually over one side of the head, nausea and vomiting. The duration of the attack is unpredictable, but it tends to follow a consistent pattern in individuals. However, only 1 in 5 migraine sufferers experiences an aura; the majority have paroxysmal headache – common migraine – that may not be confined to one side of the head.

The condition runs in families. In some individuals attacks appear to be precipitated by certain foods, or alcohol. The threshold for attacks and their frequency and severity are lowered by stress and tiredness. Sometimes an attack can be severe enough to mimic other clinical conditions, such as meningitis or subarachnoid haemorrhage, and hospital referral may be required. Complicated migraine can involve hemiplegia or hemisensory symptoms that persist beyond the resolution of the headache.

Migraine presents a dilemma because recurrent tension headaches are often labelled incorrectly as migraine and can coexist in migraine sufferers. The distinction has important implications for the choice of treatment and its outcome.

Modified essay question (MEQ)

(The instructions for the MEQ appear in the manual on page xi.)

Sandra is a 35-year-old woman with two young children, aged 2 and 4 years, living with her husband who is currently unemployed. He telephones towards the end of evening surgery requesting a visit because his wife has a severe headache and cannot stop vomiting. You can hear a child screaming in the background and her husband is quite offhand with you on the telephone. When you arrive at the house, you find the patient lying in a darkened room holding her head, with a bucket of bile beside the bed. She is a new patient so unfortunately there are no records. Around the house are full ash trays, dried food on unwashed dishes, half empty fish and chip wrappers, and a child dressed in just a nappy watching a video. You ask Sandra where her husband is. She says he has gone out, but she is not sure where.

1.   What should you do?

Her husband returns after you have been in the house 20 minutes. The history is suggestive of migraine and you decide to give an IM injection of 12.5 mg prochlorperazine (Stemetil). You ask to see the patient in the surgery the next morning.

2.   Why?

3. *What medications might you prescribe that the patient can keep at home, should she have an attack in the future?*

4. *Which one would you be least likely to initiate and why?*

5. *Would you consider prescribing prophylactic treatment? If so, what?*

    If not, why not?

6. *What drug should you consider withdrawing if she is taking it and why?*

7.   *What other type of migraine might it be important to consider in premenopausal women and how might you manage it?*

8.   *Several months elapse and you see Sandra on several occasions. You have tried all the medications you have listed and none has been of any benefit. You decide to try a prophylactic migraine preparation. Can you list the options?*

9. *Sandra admits to being tearful a lot of the time, having a poor appetite, loss of libido, mood swings and loss of concentration. What clinical condition do you suspect and which medication from those you have listed would be most appropriate?*

10. *Some years later Sandra consults very regularly with her daughter who is now aged 8 years. She complains of recurrent abdominal pain, but you can find no abnormality on examination. What might be wrong with her daughter, and why?*

MEQ answers

(Numbers in brackets refer to the marks you would receive in the MRCGP examination for each part of the answer you mention. Please total your own score to provide self-assessment.)

1. Make an assessment:
    Take a history (1)
    Examine the patient (1): exclude an acute viral infection (1); exclude meningitis (1); exclude an acute neurological event (1); exclude an acute abdomen (1).
    Provide treatment/administer an anti-emetic (2)
    Organize for someone to observe the patient (and the children), such as a neighbour or relative (2)
    Review the patient by visit or telephone (2).
    Consider referral to another member of the primary care team regarding social circumstances (1)

Comment

It is clear that orally-administered treatment would be inappropriate. Prochlorperazine is one of several alternative anti-emetic drugs (including chlorpromazine, metoclopramide and domperidone) that should relieve nausea and vomiting. If this is migraine, they may also bring the attack to a speedier conclusion. Domperidone has no injectable formulation but can, like chlorpromazine and prochlorperazine, be administered rectally as a suppository. All these drugs can have adverse effects on extrapyramidal function, although domperidone is least likely to do so because of its limited ability to cross the blood-brain barrier.

2. To build up a working doctor-patient relationship (1).
    To identify problems that may have precipitated her migraine and to see whether other social input can be provided (2).
    To gain a clearer history and confirm or refute the diagnosis of migraine (2).
    To provide the patient with medication should she have a further attack like this and to explain when and how it should be taken (2).

Comment

Establishing good rapport is a vital step in providing migraine sufferers with the reassurance that this alarming condition is essentially benign, and in helping them to manage future attacks with confidence.

3. Many possibilities include - Paramax (paracetamol and metoclopramide) (1), Migraleve (buclizine, paracetamol and codeine) (1), Migravess (aspirin and metoclopramide) (1), ergotamine (Migril) (1), sumatriptan (Imigran) (1), others (3)

Comment

Drugs suitable for use in an acute attack of migraine fall into three categories: analgesics, with or without anti-emetics; ergot derivatives; and sumatriptan.

Aspirin, paracetamol, or a non-steroidal anti-inflammatory drug, such as ibuprofen or naproxen, taken at the onset of the symptoms and repeated, if necessary, every 4 hours (keeping within the recommended daily maximum) will suffice to abort or relieve headache. Auras, when they occur, last some 20-40 minutes, and some patients with classic migraine experience a further interval of at least 10 minutes before the headache begins. This much warning affords time for an oral analgesic to traverse the stomach before gastric emptying starts to slow. Once the headache begins, it is best to give aspirin or paracetamol combined with metoclopramide to facilitate gastric emptying and allow the analgesic to be absorbed (buclizine and cyclizine, though anti-emetic, have no effect on gastric emptying). After the appearance of nausea or vomiting, analgesia can be given rectally (e.g., paracetamol, diclofenac, or indomethacin suppositories). Minor opioids, such as propoxyphene and codeine, are no more effective than simple analgesics in the management of acute attacks of migraine and may aggravate other symptoms, such as nausea and lethargy.

Ergotamine and dihydroergotamine are vasoconstrictor agents with poor and unpredictable bioavailability after an oral dose. They relieve headache in 50% of patients but can exacerbate nausea and vomiting. They should be avoided in patients with hypertension, or atheromatous disease of the coronary or peripheral arteries. Ergotamine is most easily administered sublingually or by inhalation, but is also formulated with caffeine as a suppository; dihydroergotamine, which has fewer unwanted effects than ergotamine, can be given only by injection.

Sumatriptan is a highly selective serotonin ($5-HT_{1d}$) agonist that constricts cerebral blood vessels and redistributes cerebral blood flow. Given by subcutaneous injection, it relieves headache within an hour in almost 3 out of 4 patients. After an oral dose, 2 out of 3 patients experience relief which occurs later and is less pronounced than after injection, but which exceeds the response to oral ergotamine, or to aspirin with metoclopramide. A further dose may be necessary if headache recurs within 24 hours. Sumatriptan, especially when given by injection, can give rise to a feeling of transient warmth, tingling and dizziness. It has also caused tightness in the chest and neck, the pathogenesis of which is unclear; on occasions, this has been accompanied by ECG changes, especially in patients with Prinzmetal angina. Sumatriptan should not be given to such patients, or to those with ischaemic heart disease or uncontrolled hypertension.

4. Sumatriptan: expensive (1); long-term unwanted effects not certain (1).

Comment

Sumatriptan is much the most expensive alternative and has the shortest safety record. It should be reserved for those who do not respond adequately to more established remedies.

5. Not at this stage, wait until the pattern of attacks is clear and they are occurring at least twice a month (2).

6. Any combined oral contraceptive if symptoms started following its initiation (2). These preparations can increase the frequency of attacks of migraine and predispose to complicated migraine leading to permanent clinical sequelae (2).

7. Menstrual migraine (2). This occurs within 48 hours of the onset of menstruation and may be prevented by a monthly 10 day course of a preventive agent (see below) starting one week before the period is due (2).

8. Propranolol (1).
    Pizotifen (1).
    Cyproheptadine (1).
    Tricyclic antidepressants (1).
    Calcium channel blockers (1).

Comment

Drugs that are effective in preventing attacks of migraine include beta-adrenoceptor blockers, serotonin antagonists, amitriptyline, and calcium channel blockers.

Beta-blockers reduce the frequency of attacks in 60% of patients, especially where stress is a frequent trigger. Many agents are equally effective and the mode of action is not understood. The usual contraindications apply.

Serotonin antagonists are effective in 2 out of 3 patients. Pizotifen and cyproheptadine (which is primarily an antihistamine) are most commonly used but tend to stimulate appetite and lead to weight gain, and may cause drowsiness. Methysergide is the most effective preventive agent but prolonged treatment is associated with retroperitoneal, pleural and cardiac fibrosis.

Amitriptyline, which inhibits serotonin reuptake, has effects, often at low dosage, that are independent of its effects on mood. It is not known whether other tricyclic antidepressants or selective serotonin reuptake inhibitors (SSRIs) are equally effective. Amitriptyline is not licensed for use in the management of migraine.

Calcium channel blockers, such as nifedipine or nimodipine, have not proved consistently effective in clinical trials. They may decrease the frequency of attacks after several months of treatment, but have little effect on severity.

9. Depression (2).
    A tricyclic antidepressant (2).

10. Abdominal migraine which may later become classical migraine (2).
    When migraine is familial, it often presents in childhood as abdominal pain (1).

(Total available marks = 52.)

Further reading

Bateman, D.N. (1993). Sumatriptan. *Lancet*, **341**, 221–224.
Blau, J.N. (1992). The challenge of unexplained diseases: migraine. *J. Roy. Soc. Med.*, **85(10)**, 593–594.
Lance, J.W. (1992). Treatment of migraine. *Lancet*, **339**, 1207–1209.
Macgregor, E.A. (1993). Prescribing for migraine. *Prescribers' Journal*, **33**, 50–58.
Pearce, J.M.S. (1992). Headaches. *Med. Internat.* **98**, 4086–4091.
Welch, K.M.A. (1993). Drug therapy of migraine. *N. Engl. J. Med.*, **329**, 1476–1483.

Multiple choice questions (MCQs)

(The following four statements are each followed by five answers. Please indicate whether each is true or false.)

1. **The following drugs are used to treat acute migraine:**

   a) Sumatriptan.
   b) Propranolol.
   c) Amitriptyline.
   d) Ergotamine.
   e) Paracetamol.

2. **Migraine sufferers with known ischaemic heart disease should avoid:**

   a) Soluble aspirin.
   b) Sumatriptan.
   c) Ibuprofen.
   d) Amitriptyline.
   e) Paracetamol.

3. **Symptoms of common migraine are:**

   a) Flashing lights.
   b) Abdominal pain.
   c) Diarrhoea.
   d) Vomiting.
   e) Headache with photophobia.

4. **Extrapyramidal side-effects occur with:**

   a) Soluble aspirin.
   b) Sumatriptan.
   c) Prochlorperazine.
   d) Paracetamol.
   e) Metoclopramide.

Answers overleaf

MCQ answers

(A maximum total of 20 marks are available.)

1. T,F,F,T,T.
2. F,T,F,T,F.
3. F,F,F,F,T.
4. F,F,T,F,T.

10

Thrombosis – prevention and treatment

Anticoagulation is the process by which clotting of the blood is hindered. It may be clinically indicated to prevent thrombosis *de novo*, or the extension of a clot once thrombosis has occurred, in a vein, an artery or the heart.

Two oral anticoagulants are available for use in the UK. Warfarin and phenindione both reduce clotting factor synthesis by inhibiting the activity of Vitamin K. Of the two, warfarin is much more commonly used as it has fewer unwanted effects. The onset of effect depends on the size of the initial dose but it normally takes more than 48 hours for warfarin to achieve its desired effect on coagulation. After withdrawal of treatment, coagulation returns to normal over several days.

Anticoagulant therapy presents a classical therapeutic dilemma, because of the increased risk of inducing haemorrhage as coagulation is reduced. The potential therapeutic advantages must be seen to outweigh the risks before warfarin is prescribed.

Modified essay question (MEQ)

(The instructions for the MEQ appear in the manual on page xi.)

Andrew is a 42-year-old accountant who lives in the UK, but travels regularly to the USA. He attends the surgery having just returned from New York on a transatlantic flight complaining of pain in his left calf. (He has been previously fit and well.) Examination reveals a swollen left calf whose circumference is 3 cm greater than that of the right calf. It is warm, tense and tender.

1.   Which differential diagnoses might you consider?

2.   Assume that you are a GP on the Isle of Skye with the facilities of a local GP-run cottage hospital. What therapeutic options are available?

3. Which one might you choose in Andrew's case and why?
    (Assume that you have explained to the patient the potential
    benefits of hospital treatment. However, he has opted to stay at
    home in view of the distance to the nearest district general
    hospital.)

4. As it happens, you ring the nearest consultant physician in
    Inverness and he suggests anticoagulation with low molecular
    weight heparin and warfarin. How would you initiate this
    therapy and subsequently monitor its effect? What
    contraindications might there be to the use of warfarin?

5. *After 3 weeks there has been a marked improvement in his clinical signs. However, his blood results vary greatly and he has a recurrence of a subconjunctival haemorrhage. Why might this be?*

After a further 3 weeks, you later learn from Andrew's wife, Margaret, that her husband binge drinks whisky, particularly when he is away from home, and regularly suffers indigestion. You next see Andrew a week later on a Friday evening, because his blood results show that he is over-anticoagulated (INR (International Normalized Ratio) > 5.4). He is also complaining of waking with epigastric pain in the early hours of the morning.

6. *What would be your management of Andrew now?*

After a further 2 weeks, Andrew is much improved clinically and asks if he is fit to go to New York the following week.

7. *What do you advise?*

Six months after ceasing warfarin, Andrew presents to the cottage hospital with an undisplaced fracture of his lateral malleolus. His ankle is very swollen and he has difficulty weight-bearing. You have facilities to apply a plaster of Paris.

8. *What would you advise?*

Twenty-five years later, Andrew (now aged 67 years), comes to you for a routine medical examination for life insurance. A few months earlier, while on holiday abroad, he had a transient episode of blindness in one eye lasting 2–3 hours, from which he recovered completely. You notice that his pulse is irregularly irregular and the electrocardiograph (ECG) shows atrial fibrillation with a ventricular rate of 80/min and a radial pulse rate of 72/min. His blood pressure is 150/80 mmHg. He is completely asymptomatic, apart from increasing dyspnoea when he walks more than half a mile on the level.

9. Draw up a management plan and indicate what advice you might give Andrew regarding treatment, assuming that he has read widely on the subject? (He says that he stopped drinking alcohol 6 months ago as he felt he had developed a drink problem.)

10. If you were treating Andrew for a recurrent duodenal ulcer would this alter your management?

11. *If you were having difficulty controlling Andrew's high blood pressure would this affect your management? (Imagine his BP is consistently 180/110 mmHg.)*

Three years later Andrew dies unexpectedly and suddenly in New York while on business. Autopsy confirms the cause of death as bleeding oesophageal varices. His wife, Margaret, is very distressed; she believes that his therapy may have resulted in his death.

12. *What might you say to her?*

MEQ answers

(Numbers in brackets refer to the marks you would receive in the MRCGP examination for each part of the answer you mention. Please total your own score to provide self-assessment.)

1. Deep venous thrombosis. (DVT) (2).
    Muscle tear (1).
    Cellulitis (1).
    Phlebitis of pre-existing varicose veins (1).
    Previous injury or previous thrombosis (1).
    Ruptured Baker's cyst. (1).

Comment

It is tempting to associate the occurrence of venous thrombosis with a long period spent sitting with the legs dependent, though there is no sound evidence for a causal relationship.

2. Conservative management including TED stocking (2).
    Anticoagulate with warfarin or subcutaneous heparin, or both – without confirming the diagnosis (3).
    Confirm a calf vein DVT with a venogram (1).
    Exclude thigh extension with a Doppler if available (1).

Comment

The diagnosis of a calf vein thrombosis at the bedside is unreliable. Venography, the ultimate investigation,[1] confirms the clinical suspicion in no more than 1 in 3 patients. Duplex B-mode ultrasound, which combines real-time ultrasound imaging and Doppler flow studies, is reliable in the detection of femoral and/or popliteal vein thrombosis but is unable to detect a thrombus that does not extend above the knee.[2]

If venous thrombosis is confined to the calf, the risk of pulmonary embolism is $< 1\%$ and anticoagulation is unnecessary. However, 1 in 5 calf vein thromboses will extend during the next 10–14 days to the femoral vein, increasing the risk of embolism to around 50%.[3] Ideally, if anticoagulation is withheld, the ultrasound scan should be repeated at intervals for 2 weeks to identify those at increased risk.

3. Commence both heparin and warfarin (assuming there are no contraindications) (3).
    Confident that he has a DVT clinically (1).
    Investigative facilities not available on Skye (1).
    Patient prefers this option (1).
    Treatment relatively easy to monitor (1).

4. Start daily subcutaneous injections of low molecular weight (LMW) heparin (e.g., dalteparin 200 u/kg, to maximum 18,000 u/day) and continue for at least 5 days and until the effect of warfarin given concurrently is within the target range and stable. It is not necessary to monitor the effect of LMW heparin (3). Ideally, the International Normalized Ratio (INR) should be determined before warfarin is given (2). If this is less than 1.4, give a loading dose of warfarin (10 mg daily for 2 days), then repeat the INR (5). Take the blood sample 16 hours after the second dose and then use the dosage guidance table to aid selection of the third dose. Repeat INR the following day and use the table to guide selection of the fourth dose, which should be very close to the eventual maintenance dose (2).
    Through regular blood testing and dose adjustment the INR should be maintained between 2 and 3. (3)
    Contraindications to anticoagulation: Severe hypertension; peptic ulcer; bacterial endocarditis; (pregnancy in women) (4).

Comment

LMW heparin is fractionated. Compared with unfractionated heparin it has a longer half-life and its response is more predictable, allowing a single fixed daily dose to be given without the need for laboratory monitoring. LMW heparin appears to be more effective in preventing recurrence, and less likely to cause major bleeding, than unfractionated heparin.[4]

The INR expresses the prothrombin time relative to an international standard. A dosage guidance table is available and is based on sound experimental work,[5] but the use of this table requires careful timing of the blood sample for INR in relation to the preceding dose. For example, if initial doses are taken at between 5.00 and 7.00 pm, the blood sample should be drawn between 9.00 and 11.00 am the following day, so that the result is available in good time for a decision to be made about the next dose.

Table 10.1   Warfarin dosage guidance table

Day 2 (16 hr after first 10 mg dose)	
INR	Warfarin dose (mg)
< 1.8	10.0
1.8	1.0
> 1.8	0.5

Day 3 (16 hr after second dose)	
INR	Warfarin dose (mg)
< 2.0	10.0
2.0–2.1	5.0
2.2–2.3	4.5
2.4–2.5	4.0
2.6–2.7	3.5
2.8–2.9	3.0
3.0–3.1	2.5
3.2–3.3	2.0
3.4	1.5
3.5	1.0
3.6–4.0	0.5
> 4.0	0

Day 4 (16 hr after third dose)	
INR	Warfarin dose (mg)
< 1.4	> 8.0
1.4	8.0
1.5	7.5
1.6–1.7	7.0
1.8	6.5
1.9	6.0
2.0–2.1	5.5
2.2–2.3	5.0
2.4–2.6	4.5
2.7–3.0	4.0
3.1–3.5	3.5
3.6–4.0	3.0
4.1–4.5	0 – give 2 mg from day 5
> 4.5	0 – give 1 mg from day 6

A target range of 2.0–3.0 for INR is adequate for all patients with acute venous thromboembolism except those in whom thromboembolism has recurred while the INR was already within this target range, in which case a higher range (3.0–4.5) is recommended. This higher range is also used for patients with arterial disease, including myocardial infarction, or with mechanical prosthetic heart valves.[6]

5. Is the patient taking other drugs intermittently, e.g., co-prox-amol, macrolides, cimetidine, omeprazole, ciprofloxacin or co-trimoxazole? (These may inhibit warfarin metabolism) (7).
Is the patient drinking large amounts of alcohol? (1).
Is there an underlying, undiagnosed illness? (1).
Is there a variation in diet, e.g., use of salads? (1).

Comment

The list of drugs that enhance the effect of warfarin is not comprehensive. Consult the British National Formulary (Appendix 1) for more detail. Co-proxamol contains dextro-propoxyphene, and macrolides include erythromycin and clarithromycin, all of which can inhibit the metabolism of warfarin.

Underlying illnesses that might cause variation in sensitivity to warfarin include disease of the gastrointestinal tract (affecting warfarin absorption), liver (affecting clotting factor synthesis or warfarin metabolism), or heart failure which compromises blood flow to vital organs.

Salad ingredients contain larger amounts of vitamin K than do other foodstuffs. In patients taking lifelong warfarin, it is common to see a seasonal fall in INR during the summer, necessitating higher warfarin dosage, and a converse change in the autumn. Those taking oral anticoagulants should maintain as consistent a diet as possible.

6. (a) After 6 weeks of anticoagulation following a DVT associated with a period of venous stasis the risk of haemorrhage is probably greater than the risk of embolism (1). In his case, warfarin should now be discontinued (2).
(b) Assume he may have a duodenal ulcer and start ulcer-healing therapy (2), remembering that both cimetidine (1) and omeprazole (1) may enhance warfarin's anticoagulant effect during the withdrawal phase.

Plan:

Organize an endoscopy or barium meal (1).

Advise Andrew to eat regular meals, to stop smoking (if he smokes) and to reduce his alcohol intake (4).

Comment

Assuming the DVT in this case was related to the transatlantic flight, the risk of recurrence after 6 weeks should be similar to that seen in non-elderly patients with thromboembolism occurring shortly after elective surgery, in whom six weeks of anticoagulation is now believed to be sufficient.[7] In the absence of overt bleeding, there is no need to take any therapeutic action beyond stopping warfarin. Guidance on the management of symptomatic overanti-coagulation is available elsewhere.[8]

7. He is now at no greater increased risk of a recurrent DVT than he will be in, say, a year's time (1). Good advice would be to wear TED stockings during a flight and to keep dorsi-flexing his ankles (2), and to stand up regularly and walk up and down the aisle if the cabin signs permit (1). If he was very worried, subcutaneous heparin might be considered (1).

Comment

Some airlines advise passengers aged over 55 years to wear anti-embolism stockings routinely on long haul flights and it seems a reasonable precaution in this case. Whereas aspirin reduces the incidence of venous thromboembolism in patients undergoing elective surgery and in immobilized medical patients, if taken for 1–3 weeks postoperatively or during the period of immobilization,[9] there are no data on its use by people at high risk travelling by air. However, one might reasonably advise the use of low dose aspirin under these circumstances provided there were no contra-indications.

8. Apply a plaster of Paris (1).
Encourage him to keep as mobile as possible (1).
Review if ankle pain worsens or other new symptoms occur (2).
Consider prophylactic anticoagulation whilst he has a plaster (1), assuming he has no evidence of peptic ulceration (1). (Suggest subcutaneous heparin 5000 u twice daily.)

9.   Exclude hyperthyroidism (1). Explain that he is at increased risk of a stroke (1), and the ways in which this can be prevented (1). Consider treatment with a maintenance dose of warfarin (say, 3 mg), monitored with weekly INRs (2). Raise or lower the daily dose by 1 mg to achieve INR between 2 and 3 (1). Arrange a fasting lipid screen (1).
Ask if he is still suffering indigestion (1).
If he smokes advise him to stop (1).

Comment

Patients aged 65 – 74 years with atrial fibrillation but no valvular abnormality of the heart are 4 times more likely to have a stroke than are those in sinus rhythm. This risk is increased another three-fold if they have already sustained a stroke, a transient cerebral ischaemic attack, or any other form of arterial thromboembolism. Anticoagulation with warfarin reduces this twelvefold overall increased risk by two thirds, aspirin by one third.[10] The risk of arterial thromboembolism is unaffected by a history of venous thromboembolism.

Although arterial thromboembolism will occur in one third of untreated patients with atrial fibrillation during the first 6 months after the appearance of the abnormal rhythm, the establishment of effective anticoagulation is not an urgent matter. It is not necessary to begin with a loading dose, and this allows the general practitioner to initiate treatment much more safely. Once INR is stable within the target range, it will not need to be checked more often than every 8–12 weeks unless there is a change in the patient's medical condition or drug therapy.

10.   You would be reluctant to prescribe warfarin until the ulcer has healed, because of the increased risk of haemorrhage (2). Arrange endoscopy to confirm healing prior to anticoagulation (1).
Consider detection and eradication of *Helicobacter pylori* to minimize the risk of recurrence (2).

Comment

The presence of active peptic ulceration is a contraindication to treatment with warfarin. To assess the balance of benefit and risk, only endoscopy can distinguish active ulceration reliably. If there is an ulcer, endoscopy also provides the opportunity for gastric mucosal biopsy material to be tested for the presence of Campylobacter-like organisms (CLO), to confirm or exclude infection with *H. pylori*, although this can also be done using an isotope-labelled urea breath test or by detecting antibodies in the blood. Warfarin should not be introduced until the ulcer has healed.

11. Defer warfarin therapy until his hypertension is controlled, because of the increased risk of cerebral haemorrhage (2).

Comment

Uncontrolled hypertension is a contraindication to anticoagulation.

12. You were surprised and sorry to hear her news (2).
     You explain that this could happen to anyone (1) and warfarin may have contributed to his death by increasing the severity of bleeding, but at the time treatment began there was no reason to believe that this would happen and the anticipated benefit outweighed the risk (2).
     As delicately as possible raise the subject of alcohol (1).
     Arrange to see Margaret again (1).
     Other relevant ideas (2).

(Total available marks = 98.)

References

1. Ramsay, L.E. (1983). Impact of venography on the diagnosis and management of deep vein thrombosis. *Br. Med. J.*, **286**, 698–699.
2. Editorial. (1989). Diagnosis of deep-vein thrombosis. *Lancet*, **ii**, 23–24.
3. Hull, R.D. (1989). Pulmonary embolism and venous thrombosis. *Med. Internat.*, **69**, 2877–2883.
4. Ginsberg, J.S. (1996). Management of venous thromboembolism. *N. Engl. J. Med.*, **335**, 1816–1828.
5. Fennerty, A. *et al.* (1984). Flexible induction dose regimen for warfarin and prediction of maintenance dose. *Br. Med. J*, **288**, 1268–1270.
6. *British National Formulary* No. 33 (March 1997), 108.
7. Hirsh, J. (1995). The optimal duration of anticoagulant therapy for venous thrombosis. *New. Engl. J. Med*, **332**, 1710–1711.
8. Routledge, P.A. (1993). Management of bleeding induced by oral anticoagulants. *Prescribers' Journal*, **33**, 59–63.
9. Antiplatelet Trialists' Collaboration (1994). Collaborative overview of randomised trials of antiplatelet therapy - III: reduction in venous thrombosis and pulmonary embolism by antiplatelet prophylaxis among surgical and medical patients. *Br. Med. J*, **308**, 235–246.
10. Lip, G.Y.H., Lowe, G.D.O. (1996). ABC of Atrial Fibrillation: antithrombotic treatment for atrial fibrillation. *Br. Med. J.*, **312**, 45–48.

Multiple choice questions (MCQs)

(The following four statements are each followed by five answers. Please indicate whether each is true or false.)

1. **The following are anticoagulants:**

   a) Warfarin.
   b) Heparin.
   c) Aspirin.
   d) Phenindione.
   e) Quinine.

2. **It is inadvisable to prescribe the following for a patient taking warfarin:**

   a) Ranitidine.
   b) Aspirin.
   c) Thyroxine.
   d) Erythromycin.
   e) Co-proxamol.

3. **The following statements about anticoagulation are true:**

   a) After a single DVT, warfarin should be taken indefinitely.
   b) After a single pulmonary embolism, warfarin should be taken indefinitely.
   c) Warfarin is the only drug that reduces the incidence of stroke in patients with atrial fibrillation.
   d) Patients who have had a DVT should not travel by air.
   e) Venous thrombosis confined to the calf veins is an indication for anticoagulation.

4. **If a patient taking warfarin has an INR of 7, but is asymptomatic:**

   a) Reduce daily dose of warfarin by 1 mg.
   b) Withhold warfarin for 1 to 2 days and then review.
   c) Give vitamin K, 500 micrograms IV.
   d) Stop warfarin and give vitamin K, 5 mg IV.
   e) Request urgent admission to hospital.

Answers overleaf

MCQ answers

(A maximum total of 20 marks are available)

1. T,T,F,T,F.
2. F,T,F,T,F.
3. F,F,F,F,F.
4. F,T,F,F,F.